Social Care with African Families in the UK

This imp   text promotes understanding of the complexities and diversities of   family life. It stimulates creative thinking about how social care pro   als can develop meaningful relationships and engage confidently a   ectively with African families they encounter within work contexts

The b   will help students and professionals to develop specific knowledge ar   lls for working with African families, including refugees, asylum   s, new and settled immigrants and people of dual heritage. Whilst h   ighting differences in terms of practices across the continent, the com   threads and shared identities of these families can provide the building   cks for new and relevant knowledge which then inform anti-oppressi   ractice.

Issues   ch as child discipline, officialdom, roles and responsibilities within tl   family, image and identity, and the perception of others are discussed in   hapters covering:

- economic and social pressures
- family structures
- marriage patterns/partnerships
- faith and spirituality
- mortality and death.

WINCHESTER
UNIVERSITY OF

THE LIBRARY
WITHDRAWN FROM

Containing numerous illustrative examples, this accessible text will be useful to all social work and social care students.

Viola Nzira is a lecturer in the School of Health and Social Care, University of Reading, UK.

KA 0355040 6

D0322418

Social Care with African Families in the UK

Viola Nzira

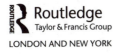

Routledge
Taylor & Francis Group

LONDON AND NEW YORK

UNIVERSITY OF WINCHESTER
LIBRARY

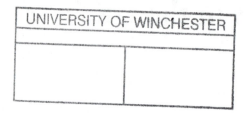

First published 2011
by Routledge
2 Park Square, Milton Park, Abingdon, Oxon OX14 4RN

Simultaneously published in the USA and Canada
by Routledge
270 Madison Avenue, New York, NY 10016

Routledge is an imprint of the Taylor & Francis Group, an informa business

© 2011 Viola Nzira

Typeset in Sabon by Wearset Ltd, Boldon, Tyne and Wear
Printed and bound in Great Britain by TJ International, Padstow, Cornwall

All rights reserved. No part of this book may be reprinted or
reproduced or utilized in any form or by any electronic, mechanical
or other means, now known or hereafter invented, including
photocopying and recording, or in any information storage or
retrieval system, without permission in writing from the publishers.

British Library Cataloguing in Publication Data
A catalogue record for this book is available from the British Library

Library of Congress Cataloging-in-Publication Data
Nzira, Viola.
Social care with African families in the UK / Viola Nzira.
p.cm.

1. Social service–Great Britain. 2. Africans–Services for–Great
Britain. 3. Africans–Great Britain–Social conditions. 4. Social work
with minorities–Great Britain. 5. Intercultural communication–Great
Britain. I. Title.

[DNLM: 1. Community Health Services–Africa South of the Sahara.
2. Community Health Services–Great Britain. 3. Social Work–Africa
South of the Sahara. 4. Social Work–Great Britain. 5. African
Continental Ancestry Group–Africa South of the Sahara. 6. African
Continental Ancestry Group–Great Britain. 7. Cross-Cultural
Comparison–Africa South of the Sahara. 8. Cross-Cultural
Comparison–Great Britain. 9. Public Policy–Africa South of the
Sahara. 10. Public Policy–Great Britain. 11. Socioeconomic Factors–
Africa South of the Sahara. 12. Socioeconomic Factors–Great Britain.
WA 546 FA1 N999s 2011]
HV245.N95 2011
362.84'96041–dc22

2010013213

ISBN13: 978-0-415-48293-6 (hbk)
ISBN13: 978-0-415-48294-3 (pbk)
ISBN13: 978-0-203-84208-9 (ebk)

Contents

Tables

Preface

What qualifies me to write a book on social care with African families?

Accident of birth, because, I was born and raised in Africa south of the Sahara, and migrated to the United Kingdom for study and work, and therefore have first hand experience of being an immigrant and raising an African family in the UK.

This background has sustained my interest and forced me to create some space for reflection, research and documenting thoughts, ideas and some suggestions for consideration by those who come into contact with African families within social care settings.

Why this book?

The African population in the UK is on the increase, and yet sourcing relevant up to date material specific to African families packaged in a coherent format to support my teaching has been difficult; hence the motivation to learn through writing this book with a view to establish those aspects that might be specific to Africans as an ethnic group as well as aiming to make a small contribution to the limited body of knowledge on social care with African families.

In preparing for, and writing this book, I have been influenced a great deal by an African childhood and adult life and professional work experiences in the UK, as well as extensive travel opportunities across Africa south of the Sahara for leisure, research and consultancy. Employment and voluntary work opportunities within the UK have included community work, public sector administration, health care clinical practice and management and, more recently, academic work specializing in social policy and public sector management. All these lived experiences, African ethnic background and gender have taught me what I know, and shaped my writing style and my suggestions for the way in which a black-African perspective could inform social care practice. However, it is important to acknowledge at the outset that the act of knowing is an extremely complex endeavour; not only do different human beings know different things, bringing different values, beliefs and perceptions to what they know and how they know it, but the act of knowing and what is known are often irredeemably fused. Knowing is itself the problematic (Oakley 2000:291).

The fusion of the act of knowing and what is known has informed the themes selected for attention, such as, the inclusion of literature for review, a questionnaire survey of African students, analysis of results and the subsequent discussion around each theme. This self-disclosure is intended to address issues of knowledge validation and to enable the expert reader to have a frame of reference for assessing and critiquing that which has been narrated.

According to James and Sharpley-Whiting (2000:187), two political criteria influence the knowledge validation process. First, knowledge claims must be evaluated by a community of experts whose members represent the standpoints of the groups from which they originate. Second, each community of experts must maintain its credibility as defined by the larger group in which it is situated and from which it draws its basic, taken for granted knowledge. In relation to this book, the community of experts would include African families living in the UK, social care students and practitioners who made contributions towards the book, as well as those who judge themselves suitably qualified to be part of a community of experts on African family life and possess the essential requirements deemed relevant for giving critical feedback on social care professional practice and academic writing that supports student learning. The key features of the book are:

- African cultural traditions,
- diversity of African families to reflect the size of the continent,
- strengths and weaknesses of different family forms,
- impact of visibility by colour on self-worth and self-esteem,
- applicability of ideas emerging from the discussion to social care practice.

Acknowledgements

Thanks to all the African social work students at the University of Reading, past and present whom I have taught over the years and for their support during the preparation of this book. They did so by their engagement in my lectures and completing a survey questionnaire about African families. Thanks to post-qualifying social work managers who shared with me during lectures the complex realities of managing social care services for diverse populations. It has been a privilege to work with both sets of students.

Introduction

The book is primarily intended for use on further and undergraduate level courses of training for social care students and their supervisors. The materials included are intended to promote an understanding of the complexities and diversities of African family life and to stimulate creative thinking about how social care practitioners can develop meaningful relationships and engage effectively with African families they encounter within work contexts. This is increasing in importance because the numbers of black African people resident in the UK and whose origins are in Africa south of the Sahara are on the increase, due in part to chronic economic dislocations in some of the former British colonies, and it is therefore likely that social care practitioners will come into contact with African families, among which, some will be asylum seekers and/or refugees. For asylum seekers and refugees, it is reported that some social workers do express concerns and at times question their ability to deal satisfactorily with culturally complex cases (Okitikpi and Aymer 2003). Apart from asylum seekers and/or refugees, it has been reported that some white workers do not possess the skills and experience to work effectively with black and minority ethnic families, and therefore hesitated in making intervention decisions; and that some white managers were unable to provide direction to black and minority ethnic workers (Butt 2006).

Additionally, the publicity that resulted from the death of Victoria Climbie and police investigations into possible ritual assaults and killings within African communities suggests the need to single out African families, as a group, for attention, while acknowledging that this group is likely to share similar experiences of discrimination and disadvantage when using social care services. It is also necessary and significant to acknowledge that, while important, these publicized cases of child abuse within the African community do not represent the reality of the experience of most African families. There are other realities of relevance and importance and worthy of note. Some of these include, for example, the daily struggles to combine study, work and managing family life. The changing family composition through interracial unions brings up the realities around dual heritage issues, and the lived experience of African children in local authority care.

Some of these children will have specific needs due to their African and European heritage (Chand 2008, Bernard and Gupta 2008, Barn 2006, Olumide 2002).

On dual heritage issues, Ifekwunigwe's (1999) research about scattered belongings provides a basis from which to contextualize the views of young people with African and European dual heritage background because the participants in her study articulated candidly their childhood experiences and socialization processes that were culturally influenced by dual heritage. Because these issues continue to be debated in social care academic circles, it seems therefore important to also give specific attention to this group. Not doing so would diminish the development of specific knowledge and skills that would enable social care workers to feel confident about their engagement with African families and young people with a racialized dual heritage. The African family issues selected for discussion take into account the variety of status among those who decided on the UK as their destination when they left their African country of origin. The issues take into account experiences of: settled immigrants, permit holders, new immigrants, refugees, asylum seekers as well as issues specific to children and young people of African/European dual heritage.

This selection is based on the experience and knowledge gained while providing tutorial support to students on social care practice placement and how coming into contact with such families highlighted some issues about the nature of social care services available to each family group. The students' experiences have demonstrated that in twenty-first century UK, there is still a need to emphasize the importance of anti-racist social care work as a technique for challenging identified individual prejudices and institutional discrimination. For this to happen, social care leaders and managers will have a pivotal role to play. This pivotal role is echoed by the Scottish Leadership Foundation (2005:2) as stated in its report:

> Good professional and practice leadership does exist and whilst there are many strengths from which to build, the scale of the challenges – demographic, social and political – that influence future design and delivery of services are such that the delivery of the vision set out by the 21st century review, particularly improving outcomes for service users and carers and communities, must be underpinned by enabling and empowering leadership and effective management.

If realistic change is to be achieved, there should be no room for discrimination within the process of enabling, empowering and effective delivery of services for all.

Some of these concerns were noted in my recent survey about social care with African families, and the details are available in Chapter 4, but the following statement made by a practitioner in response to the survey questions, provides a flavour of some of the concerns.

Many social workers abandon the need for anti-oppressive, anti-discriminatory practice once they complete their studies. Very often they fall prey of prejudices towards African families, including parents and children. These biases and prejudices often narrow their views of individual families, thereby making situations worse for these families than they were prior to their intervention. Managers do nothing about it.

(Practising social worker: participant (8))

In view of the expressed criticism, it would seem appropriate to remind social care practitioners that they are required by their professional body to adhere to the code of practice and to take into account that respect for persons must surely involve a willingness to take into account every aspect of a person's experience and circumstances, including their position in relation to society. And since we live in a society where a person's skin colour makes a difference to how people are treated, we can't ignore skin colour when considering people's needs. Respect for persons requires that we are not colour blind, at least in a society where racism still exists (Beckett and Maynard 2005:177). These two quotations encapsulate the key elements in terms of setting this book within the context of anti-racist and anti-oppressive social care practice.

The content of the book covers issues specific to families of African ancestry with direct connection with the region located south of the Sahara because of the common threads and shared identities that can provide the building blocks for additional relevant knowledge which can sustain and inform further development towards social justice and inclusion and avoiding oppressive practices. An obvious commonality binding African people is their colour, black, as well as having connections with relatives living in countries burdened with economic dislocation. 'There is a lot of pressure from the family at home for financial support. This, sometimes, forces Africans in the UK to take more than one job just to meet the demands of the family' (practising social worker (3)). Some of these economic hardships experienced by people in this region of Africa can be attributed to dramatic political shifts, regime failures, state corruption and bad governance (Fenton 2003). But, some argue that the legacy of colonialism and the specificity of capitalist development have had lasting negative effects on African societies (Eade 2002). States' corruption and bad governance are issues that often divide African communities based in the UK, because of the negative media portrayal of African nations that is seen by some Africans as not accurately representing reality. What is not in doubt is that most African people who selected to migrate and settle in the UK would, in part, have been influenced by the colonial past (Harden 1991). One way in which the socio-economic, political, cultural and intellectual processes in post-colonial Africa can be understood is through examining cultural dependency, as a result of education and a variety of selected research projects that served the needs of European and African academics and governments of the day in terms of colonial policy development.

> The study of African cultures served the needs of colonial occupiers, particularly in the creation of labour reservoirs and the segmentation of labour along ethnic lines. It was not meant to invigorate and energise those societies to absorb new positive elements to their own realities. This was reinforced by the colonial education system. African intellectuals were colonised. The medium of instruction became European languages, whose cultural influences cannot be underestimated.
>
> (Ishemo 2002:29)

Most African families living in the UK as part of settled communities or recent migrants have come from this background of implicit cultural dependency. Africans are here because British people went to Africa – be it, under very different circumstances – and the links between the UK and most ex-colonies remain.

Within the UK, media portrayal of the African continent in terms of its political, social, cultural and economic activities helps individuals outside the continent to build up a picture of where Africans came and are coming from. My direct involvement with African students with origins in West, Central, East and Southern Africa on social work courses over a period of eight years has provided me with helpful insights into the issues and themes that could be addressed within this book. Examples of issues of concern due to misunderstandings by non-Africans about African family life include: marriage patterns, child discipline, officialdom, roles and responsibilities within the family, image and identity and the perception of others. Some of these issues have been highlighted (Mvududu and McFadden 2001, Thiam 1986). To address these issues, while highlighting differences and commonalities in terms of practices in different countries, the book explores the following areas: family and child rearing practices, marriage patterns/partnerships, mortality and death, faith and spirituality. In addition to these areas, economic and social pressures are discussed within the context of migration, settlement and expectations from those left behind in the country of origin and attempts at full integration among those who settled in the UK as their adopted country. Social care policy and leadership within public sector organizations and the management of services provide a context for discussions.

The size of the continent dictates the diversity of patterns and forms of family life, as there can be no blueprint in this book. To quote (Stuart 1996:31), 'there is no such thing as "the family" in the sense of one accepted model of family life; instead, variety is the norm'. Illustrative examples are selected from four geographical regions – West, Central, East and Southern Africa – while acknowledging the limitations of such illustrations. Determination of selected countries for inclusion in the main discussions is based on access to relevant information, access to key informants and personal exposure during field trips undertaking research and consultancy.

The key informants are thirty-four social work students (current and former) of African ethnic origin whom I am teaching or have taught in the past during their period of study at first degree and/or masters levels.

Forty survey questionnaires were circulated to all African, former and existing social work students in 2008. All the respondents are currently living in the UK, and have first hand experience of an African upbringing in different parts of the continent. Countries of origin represented among the participants include: Cameroon, Gambia, Ghana, Kenya, Nigeria, Rwanda, Sierra Leone, South Africa, Tanzania, Uganda and Zimbabwe. The response rate was good, thirty-four out of forty questionnaires were returned and for details of the questions see the Appendix.

The results show that religion and spirituality are important to a significant number of Africans and have a bearing on how they deal with mortality and death. The main pressures on African family life result from lack of opportunities for good jobs, limiting their chances for advancement. Racial discrimination was considered to be a major factor in limiting their chances for securing good jobs. Cultural differences in child rearing practices were noted as aspects that caused real difficulties with officialdom. It would appear that roles within African households are gender specific and men remain heads of households; but adaptations are taking place, be it slowly. The desire to see African children achieve academically was highly rated because parents correlate academic achievement with improved prospects in the labour market.

In considering social care with African families, the core principles and values in social work are taken into account guided by international dimensions.

The International Federation of Social Workers' (IFSW) definition of social work provides a useful starting point and provides an anchor, because it goes beyond statutory functions and states:

> The social work profession promotes social change, problem solving in human relationships and the empowerment and liberation of people to enhance well-being utilising theories of human behaviour and social systems, social work intervenes at the points where people interact with their environments. Principles of human rights and social justice are fundamental to social work.
>
> (Lyons *et al.* 2006:3)

Within this definition, empowerment and liberation have poignancy, because supporting African families towards liberation is likely to bring measurable rewards for all concerned. Migrants take risks and do so because they are looking for a better life, therefore, are usually prepared to graft, given the opportunity.

Social care thought and professional practice ideas are considered progressively in each chapter, taking into account key elements included in the international definition of what social work is about. Specific consideration is given to the ideas relating to African social traditions and African centred worldview that refers to issues of interconnectedness of human beings spiritually, so that the human being is never an isolated individual but always the person in the community (Graham 2002:70). Attention is given to African feminism and its influence on the debates about the position of women across Africa south of the Sahara.

Chapter outlines

Chapter: 1 Africans at home and UK diaspora

The first part of Chapter 1 provides information about family life in Africa south of the Sahara, while taking into account the impact of historical events and some of the responses to those events. References are made to the current state of affairs in relation to social, cultural and economic imperatives that influence family life. Gender inequality and some of the reasons for its continuation are discussed. United Nations publications and research evidence provided by Hutson (2008), Kevane (2004), Snyder (2000) and Davidson (1984) informs much of the discussion.

The second part of Chapter 1 shifts the focus to Africans who are living in the UK, highlighting their reasons for migration and their experiences of UK based family life. Drawing on census data, relevant government information and social research evidence, the connections between African countries and the UK are highlighted. From the analysis of various studies, common threads that bind together most Africans resident in the UK are made explicit taking into account patterns of migration and settlement as well as acknowledging the dangers associated with universalizing the human experience. Issues affecting the lives of Africans are discussed, giving specific attention to education, economic activity and health and well-being.

Hall's (1997) work on culture, identity and cultural representation, provides a theoretical framework for conceptualization and discussion. Understanding where African people are located as they live their lives in terms of the process of 'becoming' as well as of 'being' is important, taking into account the traumatic colonial past as well as the recent traumatic experience of independent Africa and some of its failures. More importantly, acknowledging successes against difficult circumstances is identified so as to counteract the dominance of negativity bestowed on Africa and its peoples. Students are asked to consider evidence based practice issues and to create a research question, followed by a consideration of a possible research design. It is intended that students can be encouraged to test their understanding of the main issues about migration and identity, while identifying the gaps in knowledge which can be addressed through research. This process can assist practitioners towards gaining confidence when interacting with African families without fear of racism accusations.

Chapter 2: Social care and policy context

The discussion draws attention to political ideologies and their influence on the creation and maintenance of the welfare state. Issues relating to immigration, citizenship and welfare benefits are considered, highlighting their possible impact on Africans and their families. Poverty is explained and the role of social care practitioners in supporting poor African families is addressed.

Chapter 3: Organizational and leadership context

The ideas covered in this chapter are intended to give a prominent position to organizational and leadership practices in view of government policy about managerialism and leadership in the public sector. It is an area that is receiving a great deal of attention nationwide in view of the changing nature of the location of users of public services. The issues of diversity among users of public services and their expected involvement as active participants suggest that social care organizations and those who lead them are expected to change in response to the new demands. Where Africans as users of public services fit in is discussed and areas for further improvement are indicated.

Chapter 4: Student survey

The results from the questionnaire survey are presented and the main points to emerge are discussed, highlighting possible implications for African families and those who work with them within the social care sector.

Chapter 5: Social, cultural and economic pressures

In this chapter the common threads identified in Chapter 1 provide the basis for an exploration and discussion of African experiences within the education system, in the job market and the impact of economic activity on family life at home and abroad (UK and country of origin). Women and men's experiences are examined to illuminate areas of major differences worth noting. Liberation theory provides the basis for analysis, and from the analysis suggestions are presented in terms of effecting personal changes. In common with most young people in the UK, children within these families copy and are influenced by their parents, the schools, peers and society at large; therefore aspects relating to modelling are considered.

Potential for affective destructive conflict between cultures informs the debate and a synthesis of practice ideas is presented for consideration. Students are asked to undertake an electronic search of published information about an African country south of the Sahara that they know the least about in order to learn about family life within that country.

Chapter 6: Marriage patterns

Theoretical underpinning for this chapter is culture, from functionalism and structuralism perspectives when considering issues of cohesion and continuity, as well as the ideas around symbolism and the activities that inform the construction of everyday social reality for Africans living in the UK. Choice of function and structure as perspectives is influenced by an identified link to an established systems theoretical framework that is used extensively in the social care field around work with families.

The discussion in this chapter addresses the multiplicity of patterns and views surrounding marriage, the importance and status of bride-wealth/bride-price among those who have settled outside their countries of origin. As people integrate, are they likely to want something different? If so, can they still remain within their communities? An attempt to provide answers to these questions is made and students are directed to areas for further exploration through an activity about bride-price and implicit values that guide thought processes about the issue of bride-price.

Chapter 7: Family and child rearing practices

Analysis of social work with families using systems theory provides the basis for examining family structures and power theory to support the ideas about bargaining power within the African home. It is intended that the ideas from this chapter will show how marriage patterns affect family structures. These structures will reflect the relations of power, status and locations of those who inhabit the 'African family' as an institution. The emphasis on power focuses attention on aspects of supportive and emancipatory practices that are likely to help to produce knowledge that can inform future social care practice. Nuclear, extended and polygamous family structures and the dilemmas they each present are mapped out, taking into consideration UK legislation on marriage and immigration. The rationale for giving significant attention to marriage patterns and family life is to highlight that, while marriage is favoured by many, the reality is that 30 per cent of all families in Africa south of the Sahara are headed by female lone parents for a variety of reasons (Owen 1996, UN 2005). These women seem to get on with managing their lives and do not see themselves as victims, suggesting that this might be an area of strength that can be tapped into when considering appropriate responses to the needs of African lone parents living in the UK. Self-assessment of comprehension is encouraged through a set of questions on different family structures and values underpinning childcare practices in Africa.

African women's perspectives inform the main discussion taking into account of how this perspective deals with childcare issues. This area of social care practice can be fraught with difficulties and interventions may not be effective if the practitioners do not have a sound knowledge base about the diversity of African child rearing practices. Students are encouraged to draw on first-hand practice experience, as a basis for critiquing existing literature on approaches to childcare. The ideas about the family are further developed taking into account the mother–child nexus, which forms the core of families universally, even though having a child does not necessarily put women where they can access social resources. The ideology of domesticity, which locates women in places of motherhood, will also inform the discussion in view of the pressures to secure and retain full-time employment. All African women who migrate to the UK expect to be economically active. Such expectations from within the individual, partners, the community and the extended family abroad, place huge burdens on individual women as they try to juggle their responsibilities around motherhood and full-time employment.

Following on from the discussion about the family, the exploration further considers individual roles, responsibilities and relationships among family members in order to establish positive and negative aspects and their impact during the process of integration. The economics of marriage underpin the discussion taking into consideration the view that marriage practices vary greatly across societies and regions, as well as among people within a single region. How should social workers, confronted with such complexities, respond? A no-one-best-way approach informs attempts to formulate an answer to the question drawing on the ideas about a person centred approach as cited in the Department of Health 'Valuing People White Paper' (2002a).

Chapter 8: Religion and spirituality

This chapter addresses the role of religion, faith and spirituality among Africans living in the UK and how that role impacts on social, economic and family life. Christianity, Islam and ancestral veneration are common religious traditions within Africa. A brief account of each religion is provided supported with a commentary indicating possible implications for practice when professional practitioners come into contact with those who are active participants of specific religious denomination. The key message is about recognizing active participation and avoidance of assumptions about patterns of spirituality between, say, rural and urban dwellers. Questions are put to the reader about African religions, their importance and methods that could be used to engage African church groups as stakeholders in social care.

Chapter 9: Ageing, mortality and death

Life expectancy in most African countries is less than sixty years, suggesting that structures aimed at supporting older people would not have been a priority. It is therefore necessary in this chapter to discuss what it would mean for people of African ancestry to grow old in the UK as they face their mortality and death. Where is home? Where is the last resting place? A common tradition of repatriating the deceased to an ancestral home remains a challenge to the establishment. Theories of attachment and loss inform the discussion, so as to establish if there are Euro-centric and Afro-centric differences, and implications of those differences to social care practice. An activity invites students to answer questions on how Africans support their elders, express grief and reasons for returning to Africa after death.

Chapter 10: Negotiating and balancing the demands from two cultures

The demands from African and European cultures are explained. A discussion that follows the explanation is informed by survey results and focuses attention on issues of identity, integration and coping strategies. Emphasis is placed on the differences between adults and young people in terms of how they adjust and adapt to their new environment. A case study is included, accompanied by a set of questions about needs assessment and behaviours apparent in the case study.

Conclusion

This chapter revisits all the chapters and provides brief summaries of the main points covered and offers ideas about their relevance when supporting African families. The chapter gives prominence to the importance of managing change and the role of leadership and management in making the change happen. At individual front line practitioner level, change is also suggested around knowledge acquisitions, skills development, behaviour and attitudinal change in line with the requirements of the General Social Care Council (GSCC) codes of practice and social care professional values.

1 Africans at home and UK diaspora

This chapter will:

- provide contextual information about Africans south of the Sahara desert,
- examine the characteristics of the UK based African population from this region,
- discuss implications for policy and social care provision.

Africans south of the Sahara

In the middle of 2008 the African population south of the Sahara desert was estimated to be about 809 million, distributed over forty-three countries, from Angola to Zimbabwe when arranged in alphabetical order. Around 42 per cent of this population is below the age of fifteen suggesting continued population growth in the foreseeable future as these young Africans reach maturity and enter their reproductive phase (Population Reference Bureau and African Population Research Centre 2008). Against this expected population growth concerns about poverty continue to be a real challenge. According to Moyo (2010), Africa south of the Sahara remains the poorest region in the world, with an average per capita income of roughly US$1 a day. She suggests that the extreme poverty conditions experienced by a significant African population is likely to be around for some time unless drastic measures are taken to include a rethink on aid donations. Drawing on United Nations Human Development forecasts, she points out that Africans south of the Sahara, will account for almost one-third of world poverty by 2015. The poor living conditions and political distress resulting from dictatorship and non-democratic rule means that some Africans are likely to continue to be tempted to migrate to the West in search of a better life. From some of these African countries, some people have migrated to the UK and the figures as per the 2001 census are recorded at 478,181 people. As a proportion of the overall African population, it is evident that this figure represents a very small, but nevertheless an important, UK minority group, because most of the Africans within this group originated from former British colonies.

Geographically, Africa is an enormous landmass inhabited by people with established complex social systems of custom, habit and community life as well as having a diversity of more than 1000 languages (Davidson 1984). The size of the continent and the cultural diversity of its people suggest that Africa cannot be treated as a single entity or Africans be treated as a single branch of the human species. In an earlier publication Davidson (1961) offered a view about a different relationship that existed between Africa and Europe based on trade before colonization. He thinks that at the beginning of their connection, Africa and Europe traded and met as equals. There was acceptance of equality based on the strength and flexibility of feudal systems of state organization which governed the relations between the two continents. However, the slave trade and colonization altered the balance of power that has continued to have a negative impact due in part to economics and limited industrialization in most African countries south of the Sahara.

> On Africans the mentality of the slaving years has tended to produce a contrary effect: it has sometimes loaded Africans with a sense of inferiority and even, here and there, of guilt and shame; and this too, in one or other devious form still persist.
>
> (Davidson 1961:246)

The slave trade was followed by colonization which is viewed as the world's messiest experiment in cultural and political change that took place over a period of about twenty-five years after which the colonizers turned their authoritarian creation over to the African leaders some of whom have turned into authoritarian dictators. In recent times the indications suggest that Africa is still home to at least eleven fully autocratic regimes (Moyo 2010). Countries with such autocratic regimes include Congo, Equatorial Guinea, Eritrea, Gabon, Gambia, Mauritania, Rwanda, Sudan, Swaziland, Uganda and Zimbabwe. There is no sign that the leaders of these countries are likely to relinquish their hold on power soon.

Questions continue to be raised as to why African political leaders become dictators and refuse to give up power. Robert Mugabe is the latest leader who has been in the spotlight because he refused to concede defeat at the 2008 elections. Commentators seem perplexed about his transformation from freedom fighter to a dictator within a period of about twenty-five years. Perhaps the education system of his youth contributed to the man he became or maybe he was selective on which aspects of imperial formal education to adopt. What is important to note is that the majority of Africans who migrate to the West from countries like Zimbabwe will have been forced by circumstances beyond their control to uproot themselves in search of security and improved life opportunities. Critics of the ruthlessness and the lack of moral and ethical consideration of some African leaders infer some association with the behaviours of their colonial masters during the nineteenth and twentieth centuries. For example the British colonial, cultural and political experiment is thought to have influenced some of these leaders because the processes used did not involve ethics or consent.

> Africans were not asked whether they wanted to be guinea pigs. They were bullied into it. Europeans overwhelmed the continent in the last quarter of the nineteenth century, looking for loot. They carved it up into weirdly shaped money-making colonies, many of them landlocked, all of them administered from the top down. The colonies bore little or no relation to existing geographical or tribal boundaries.
>
> (Harden 1991:16)

With colonization, it can be argued that Africans became social hybrids because they were born into one race and brought up to live like members of another race, externally in contradiction with themselves; as such this inserted a destructive wedge between Africans and their established cultural norms and community life.

Missionaries played a part in condemning African beliefs as savage and implicitly encouraged people to accept a social hybrid status. The extent to which Africans have moved away from this hybrid status is yet to be accurately measured. There are differing views on the current state of personal development through mental liberation. The social, economic and political difficulties experienced by many African countries could in part be attributed to the hybrid status and a sense of inferiority that leads those in power to seek external support from outside Africa rather than utilizing existing knowledge within Africa to solve economic, social and political problems. Going West or going East for financial aid and military arms appears to be a preoccupation for some African leaders, reinforcing a possible state of inferiority that makes the leaders think that Africans are not capable of manufacturing goods that can be traded on the international market.

Davidson (1984:271) considers that true development is possible for Africa, and states:

> The solution for the black African continent is to know and accept the past as the crucial soil that can nourish the present: in practice, to shape models of society, patterns of community, types of development, which are appropriate to the African needs, and not to the needs of some other people in a different continent.

While the above suggestion is made by an outsider with an intense interest on Africa and its peoples and has travelled and written extensively about Africa, it must be up to Africans who must use their own genius to determine the nature of economic development. Until that happens,

Africans currently resident in the UK remain connected to their family members in Africa who are going through transition, experiencing economic hardships, while they, in the UK, grapple with their hybridized ethnic minority status.

Nangoli (1986) in his publication about his strongly held views of Africa seen through the eyes of an African man, highlights some of the problems associated with Africa's inbuilt dependence on industrial economies of Europe and North America. He is critical of the African education systems because he sees them as being inappropriate for the advancement of African societies, since the education teaches consumerism at the expense of production for international trade. Most of the manufactured goods Africa needs are imported, while Africa exports raw materials at a price determined by economically powerful nations, thereby putting its people at an economic disadvantage. The African exclusive privilege of making people in the industrialized North rich through exporting raw materials is an aspect that requires urgent attention. Nangoli (1986) offers a process that could be followed to bring about that which Africans desire as follows:

- mental decolonisation,
- rekindling the lost spirit of nationalism,
- stimulation of the desire to be free and self-reliant,
- injection of lost dynamism through visionary leadership,
- use of Africa-wide common language,
- economic cooperation among African nations,
- valuing fraternal co-existence,
- valuing individual freedoms,
- creation of African oriented systems of government,
- develop education systems appropriate to Africa's needs,
- export manufactured products not raw materials.

By following the above process Nangoli argues that Africans will reduce their collective economic dependency on the industrialized North and, as consumers, become less vulnerable because they will no longer be at the mercy of producers. The suggested process has some merit, but fails to tackle the leadership impasse in a way that would convince the majority to rise up against those leaders who continue to abuse their own people. He also fails to address the important issue of gender inequalities in African societies, even though he acknowledges that African societies are unbashfully male oriented and that men have the upper hand on matters affecting African populations. This upper hand curtails the freedoms of many women. With specific reference to South Africa, President Mandela noted that freedom cannot be achieved unless women have been emancipated from all forms of oppression (Hutson 2008). The reference to oppression suggests underutilization of African women towards economic independence for all these African nations.

Gender inequality

The African feminist position post independence and national building is that women in Africa engage in productive and reproductive labour and yet their labour remains invisible and devalued but remains indispensable to the viability of states and their economies (Adomako Ampofo *et al.* 2004). Feminism seeks to modify or transform pre-existing gender relations to allow women and men equal rights and opportunities within a particular socio-economic framework (Drew 1995). African feminist thought emphasizes the importance of context specific examination of behaviour and practice issues associated with gender subordination in order to illuminate manifestations. African feminism highlights the need to be sensitive to the social context and complexities of women's and men's lives since many cultures and identities exist in Africa and all deserve to be acknowledged and included in scholarly activities. Issues that have been raised are linked to what has been described as neo-colonial African states that have sought to retard women's basic rights. These states have done so through the re-establishment of traditional courts and statutes in the legal systems.

However, there are issues of concern that would need to be addressed if progress is to be made towards recognition of equality between the sexes in cultural economic and political spheres within each African country. These issues are noted within the following statements:

- women continue to work long hours within and outside the home,
- gender segregation within the job market,
- boys outnumber girls in education,
- male violence against women,
- subservient roles are designated to and accepted by women,
- women do not inherit land or property in most African countries,
- women's conformity and obedience,
- oppression, exploitation and discrimination against women.

These issues are not unique to Africa, but the approach to tackling them differs between the industrialized West and Africa south of the Sahara. As indicated earlier, poverty affects many families in Africa and this has serious implications for the choices women make in relation to political activism and challenging male dominance that negatively affects their lives. Women continue to conform to the social and societal norms with which they were brought up. This conformity is particularly evident in the area of gender based violence where no customary law exists to protect women against violence. It seems that the internalization of cultural norms about the right of men to control women lead many African societies to condone the physical disciplining of women and girls. The available research suggest that many African men make important economic decisions without involving women, have power over women and fail to treat women with respect (Dolan 2001, Koenig *et al.* 2003, Southern African Research and Documentation Centre (SARDC) 2000). Ending the oppression of women is culture dependent; therefore, any strategies formulated to effect change would need to be informed by positive cultural aspects so as to ensure that women's empowerment is achieved. Women would need to be prepared to take on the challenge to changing the culture and tradition of male dominance that is not conducive to the needs of twenty-first century Africa. There are some examples of successful challenges to male dominance in areas related to economic activity (Snyder 2000). Against the odds some African women are succeeding in small to medium size enterprises in some West and East African countries. There are also examples where some women have had the courage and resilience to fight back and find a way to bridge the gap between traditional tribal ways and modern twenty-first century life. One such example is that of three South African women spanning three generations. These three women worked and raised children in a culture and society where black women had hardly any rights, were daily discriminated against by apartheid and were regarded as the property of their husbands or fathers (Mathabane 1994:xiii). Through the narratives of their lived experience, it is left to the reader to note those actions that made it possible for these women to refuse to buckle under tradition, custom and oppression. It seems quite simple, but the common thread that runs through these women's narratives is the word 'no'. No to domination, no to abuse and no to subservience. They are critical of the outmoded customs and traditions that serve to stifle women's growth and strangle their dreams, preventing them from becoming equal partners of men. Recording ideas from a diversity of narratives from women's experiences of resisting oppression can inform specific areas for future research. The evidence can then be used to draw up plans for action including the style and nature of evaluation in order to assess impact.

The discussion about Africa and its people has thus far considered issues of diversity, external influences, women's subordinate status, male dominance and their implications in relation to economic activity and family relationships. The discussion provides some contextual information to enhance an understanding of family life among Africans living in the UK because it is likely that their African connections will have partly shaped their worldview and how they are likely to conduct themselves within a predominantly white European environment. The next part of the chapter deals with issues about Africans living in the UK.

Africans living in the UK

Historically, Africans have resided in Great Britain since antiquity. Very early on, Africans were few in number, but from the twentieth century onward their numbers showed a substantial increase. Initially, African men came as seafarers and settled in established ports or as students with a view to further their education, then return to their countries of origin to secure good jobs. The Africans seafarers who decided to stay came mainly from West and East Africa and settled mainly in the docklands of London, Liverpool and Cardiff (Killingray 1994). Successful companies and missionaries sponsored African students to attend British universities pre-Second World War. However the pattern of student migration changed when African British colonies gained independence during the 1960s. Some students decided not to return to their countries of origin, but to settle permanently in Britain. This was the beginning of settled African communities. The political instabilities of the 1970s and 1980s produced a new immigrant population of African refugees (Oguibe 1994). Between 1980 and 1991, 8500 Africans were granted refugee status and exceptional leave to remain (Daley 1998). According to national statistics office, between 1971 and 1991, the African population living in the UK rose from 200,025 to 478,181. At the last census in 2001, there was a slight increase to 1 per cent of the UK population. Current projections suggest that the African population will increase to 1.2 per cent by next year – 2010 (Equalities Review 2007).

Characteristics

Africans living in the UK have varied characteristics that include, for example, length of stay, country of origin, immigration status and place of residence. The majority of Africans live in London, estimated to be about 83 per cent of the UK African population due to the perceived better opportunities for employment and access to well established African community groups and societies.

The remaining percentage of this African population is found in other metropolitan cities and university towns such as Liverpool, Manchester, Birmingham, Oxford and Sheffield. Available statistics suggest that Africans are underrepresented in rural areas. This is a reverse to the situation in Africa, where the majority of the population reside in rural areas. However, Africans who manage to migrate to the West tend to be urbanites from Africa's big cities, therefore less likely to be fazed by metropolis environments per se, even though the pace of human interaction and the conduct of business activities is faster than that found in African cities. On arrival, some of the problems Africans face are linked to unemployment and/or underemployment because, without a job, social and welfare needs are unlikely to be met. This limited economic activity is not always due to lack of qualifications, as other factors play a part. For example, racism and discrimination are thought to be contributory factors, although some people might disagree.

> Among black African, qualifications do not necessarily guarantee access to the labour market. Fourteen per cent of those with qualifications are unemployed, 48 per cent of those unemployed have A levels,

39 per cent with first degree or equivalent, and 13 per cent have higher degrees.

(Daley 1998:172)

Elam and Chinouya (2000), in their study of the black African population living in the UK, focusing on four established African communities in London, namely, Ghanaian, Nigerian, Somali and Ugandan, found that there were more common experiences to all communities due to their minority status, than were differences. Social networks were considered to be essential as survival strategies enabling members of these communities to associate and to feel a sense of belonging, while they fight against poverty and forge ahead to improve their income and status. However, in this study it was noted that there are difficulties in using government data as a basis for estimating population size due to census under-recording. Population estimates can be used in a controversial manner dependent on the message intended and the target audience and scenarios of them-and-us.

This under-recording was echoed by AFRUCA (2008:5), and offered a view that the African population could be higher than government figures would indicate.

While their margin of error remains speculative, there seems to be agreement that Africans are the fastest growing ethnic minority group in the UK, overtaking African-Caribbean and other groups. Among the adult population, it may be that some individuals are in the UK illegally having decided to remain when their visas expire. Homeless African people would not be registered for census purposes and therefore excluded from the final population tally. The argument seems to be that there are more Africans living in the UK than official government statistics would suggest, but by what percentage remains a difficult question to answer. If people are in the country illegally, poverty can be a problem because they are unlikely to have recourse to public funds, receive goods and some services, therefore are unlikely to receive statutory social support due to their immigration and/or citizen status. AFRUCA, as an organization that focuses attention on safeguarding children, wishes to draw attention to the estimated rapid growth in the number of African children in the UK, showing an increase from 97,667 in 1992 to 145,677 in 2000.

This growth is significant because of the level of poverty among African families. 'As with other minority families, their level of poverty is reported to be higher than the majority white population due to higher levels of unemployment and low paid jobs' (Alcock 1997:291). Poverty is an important policy issue because poverty sustains persistent inequalities in the UK for all ethnic groups and needs to be tackled, and social care practitioners can assist in highlighting the extent of poverty among specific user groups and individual families.

While acknowledging the recent demographic changes, it is important also to recognize the point made earlier that Africans have been coming to the UK in small numbers since the nineteenth century and in significant numbers since the 1970s, initially as students to attend university and subsequently to work. More recently, the pattern of migration has changed to include Africans escaping conflict and repression, from countries such as Angola, Congo, Liberia, Sierra Leone, Somalia and Zimbabwe. Among these Africans, some entered the UK as asylum seekers or refugees and others arrived as work permit holders having secured employment in areas where opportunities existed such as schools, health and social care. Work permit holders who are economic migrants do so because they are unable to secure paid employment in their own countries or decide not to return home after completing their courses of study (Elam and Chinouya 2000).

Immigration and employment status have implications for housing. It is likely that Africans who are new to the UK would be found living on poor housing estates, supported by relatives and friends. Likewise, for individuals who have become settled and established, their housing conditions would be similar to that of the rest the population, suggesting that some people from these communities do integrate, contribute to society and achieve their goals and become role models to others, and such examples of success stories could be made public to motivate other Africans as well as to inform the rest of the population that some Africans do achieve recognized success and make measurable contribution to the UK society. In her annual article on society (Dunnell 2008) provides useful statistical analysis on diversity and different experiences in the UK. Areas of concern in relation to the African population include poverty, overrepresentation in the mental health care system and school level academic achievement being lower than the comparable white population. However, on the positive side, in view of the ageing population, Africans as a group like other ethnic minority groups have a younger age structure than the majority white population. The doubling in number of African children within a period of eight years confirms this point. Africans who migrate tend to be young adults who are trying to make it in the West and are of child bearing age, hence the noticeable increase in African child population.

Planning for this increase in the numbers of children born to African parents would ensure that their future needs are appropriately taken into account. For example, ensuring that cultural identity issues are incorporated into the way welfare services are organized and delivered would support the principles of inclusion and avoid discrimination against Africans.

Cultural representation and identity

There is a diversity of cultures among Africans living in the UK, because of the diversity of the countries of origin. The culture within each country can be viewed as shared values that determine a distinctive way of life of people of that country. Language, feelings, attachments, emotions and ideas are part of culture.

> To say two people belong to the same culture is to say that they inter-
> pret the world in roughly the same ways and can express themselves,
> their thoughts and feelings about the world, in ways which will be
> understood by each other. Thus culture depends on its participants
> interpreting meaningfully what is happening around them, and making
> sense of the world in broadly similar ways.
>
> (Hall 1997:2)

In considering the definition of culture and examining the ideas within it, it can be deduced that Africans who migrate to the UK will bring with them a variety of ways in which they make sense of the world. Their culture specific worldview will inform their approach to adaptation and integration in the new culture. Within the new culture representation con-nects with meaning and language to make culture. As part of the adapta-tion process Africans are likely to encounter stereotyping as a signifying practice central to the representation of racial difference (Hall 1997). Rep-resented as the other, the African is more likely than not to occupy a sub-ordinate and powerless position as a newcomer with a specific immigration status such as: economic migrant/asylum seeker/refugee. But it is possible to minimize the impact of negative representation of Africans by offering alternative ideas, concepts and theories that can be used to analyse cultural and ethnic differences.

Graham (2002) suggests ways of reversing stereotypes by engaging with African centred philosophy. It is a holistic approach that gives attention to values that inform and influence a particular way of being and of living. She cites the interconnectedness of all things, hence, a holistic system that encompasses spirituality, inclusiveness and interpersonal relationships. She argues that this interconnectedness makes most Africans feel that they are part of the natural environment they inhabit and are close to nature and that they readily acknowledge the value of interdependency.

Graham (2002:97) argues that the attributes of African centred world-views can be utilized by any group or individuals interested in pursuing social work approaches that insist upon spirituality, humanism, cultural recourse knowledge and human possibilities in designing effective interventions.

The human possibilities idea is an important one to consider, in relation to Africans who decide to migrate to other parts of the world, such as migrating to the industrialized West. It takes drive and inner strength among those individuals who move away from familiar environments determined to make a success of their life in a foreign country. The strength perspective has a part to play in counteracting negative represen-tations of Africans living in the UK. To successfully enter the UK requires enormous strength because of the 'hoops' that must be negotiated. A non-determined African would not make it. Acknowledging the strength within most Africans who have successfully negotiated their way into the UK, would be a good basis from which to begin the interactive process. Africans come from oral traditions, making storytelling a common occurrence (Achebe 1960). It seems therefore helpful to seriously consider adopting a strength perspective, thereby providing opportunities for Africans to 'tell' their stories, expressing hopes and fears to a respectful non-judgemental audience of professional practitioners.

From these cultural and personal stories, solutions to problems can be worked out. According to Canda (1997:86), cultural stories, narratives and myths, accounts of origins and migration, or trauma and survival may provide sources of meaning and inspiration in times of difficulty or confusion.

The strength perspective can benefit the helper and the person seeking help. Social care workers who are in a position to help can consider the views about cultural representation, African centred worldview and strength perspective and decide on possible usage as they engage with African families. It is important to do so because the evidence suggests problems still exist (Miller 2006, Nzira and Williams 2009). Among Africans living in the UK, government statistics highlight three interrelated areas for social care attention, namely, poverty, education and mental health (Dunnell 2008). In the next section the discussion focuses on these three areas.

Poverty

If the government's intention to eradicate child poverty within a decade is achieved, all children are more likely to benefit, and, if so, they might all make a contribution to society through paid employment and pensions for old age. The basis for calculating the poverty line is the income needed by a household for meeting basic needs of living. The poverty line supports the calculation of social security benefits. Poverty is the number and percentage of individuals living in households with below 60 per cent of median income (before housing costs) (Dunnell 2008). It can be argued that poor people tend to be socially excluded from mainstream society, but poverty due to unemployment is not the only aspect linked to social exclusion, as illustrated by the following definition: 'exclusion processes are dynamic and multidimensional in nature. They are linked not only to unemployment and/or low income, but also to housing conditions, levels of education and opportunities, health discrimination, citizenship and integration in the local community' (European Social Policy White Paper 1994:37, cited in Llewellyn *et al.* 2008).

Such a working definition would suggest that member countries will put in place national social policies to tackle social exclusion. In considering poverty as a contributor to social exclusion, some African families are likely to be caught up in the cycle of deprivation and find themselves living in relative poverty. While it is generally accepted that poverty is a social problem – going as far back as the Rowntree's study of 1899, which established a pattern for future studies on poverty drawing on the concept of the poverty line, a level of income at which one is deemed to be in poverty – the difficulties have been about workable solutions.

Many people, including academics, politicians and campaigners talk about the problem of poverty; and underlying their discussion is the assumption that identifying the problem provides a basis for action on which we all agree. However, people do not all agree on what the problem of poverty is, and thus, not surprisingly, the action they wish to encourage or justify is not all the same. 'Poverty is not just a state of affairs; it is an unacceptable state of affairs – it implicitly contains the question, what are we going to do about it' (Alcock 1993:3).

Within the framework of the welfare state, the answer would be adequate social security benefits for those who can demonstrate a need and are eligible to receive state support by virtue of their status as citizens of the UK. Not everyone who is resident here and is in poverty, according to the definition, can have recourse to public funds. What can social care workers do about it? Some African families may not meet the eligibility criteria as part of national immigration policy, therefore children in such poor households are likely to incur multiple forms of deprivation, at a time when their parents had wanted a better future for them, hence the reason for migration in the first place.

The impact of poverty on children is well documented and arguments have been put forward and explanations provided as to the importance for urgent government action to tackle this social problem. Some of the responses from government have included a number of initiatives such as Sure Start and pre-school education for all three and four year olds. Poverty linked to structures of society remains a major problem, and even though emancipatory social work has been successful in highlighting structural and ideological factors that perpetuate the continuation of poverty, practical workable steps are still awaited. Critics of managerialism point to the fact that social workers are spending a great deal of their time, monitoring, maintaining and supervising those most damaged by poverty (Jones 2002).

For example, it is estimated that children living in poverty are more likely to be received into local authority care (Bebbington and Miles 1989). Thoburn *et al.*'s (2005) study on child welfare services concluded that African children were almost twice as likely to be looked after by the local authority than their numbers in the population at large. Why is this the case?

Unfortunately, overall outcomes for looked after children nationally are not good. A combination of representational factors – poor, African, in care – would be a cause for concern, suggesting therefore the importance of considering other ways of looking after children in addition to existing arrangements in place. Alternative forms of care for African children in need would be worth considering, while maintaining the principle of safe-guarding children. There is further discussion on alternative approaches in Chapter 7 on child rearing practices within African communities. Investigating effectiveness of alternative arrangements for childcare would require investment in time, energy, commitment, money and above all an acceptance that other approaches have merit and should be given a chance in the interest of the children.

School performance

Supported by the idea of meritocracy, government policy on education has been about pushing for improved educational attainment for all children from all backgrounds to enable them to do well in the labour market, thereby reduce inequalities (Llewellyn *et al.* 2008). Among minority ethnic groups, it has been reported that children from African families experience a lower quality home learning environment on average than children from other ethnic groups, (Equalities Review 2007). A good home learning environment supported by a good pre-school experience is likely to lead to good educational attainment.

This is an area requiring direct parental attention, provided they are made aware of a school's expectations from parents outside the classroom. Some African parents may have come from countries with systems of education, where all required learning takes place within a structured classroom setting. The active involvement of some African parents in their children's education can be hampered by poverty, where parents take on more than one job to make ends meet for the immediate family in the UK as well as providing remittances to extended family members back home in Africa because of their interdependency cultural norm (Elam and Chinouya 2000). The intensity of pressures resulting from juggling more than one job can have an impact on the amount of quality time available to some African parents to support their children with their homework and additional learning outside the structured school environment, which may not be seen as a priority when parents are struggling to make ends meet financially. Acknowledging the realities of existence for some of the poor families would be a useful starting point in engaging the parents towards an understanding of the way in which education and social care systems function in the UK. Informed parents are likely to seek ways to support their children, once they become aware of the level and quality of input expected from home. For those parents who are not familiar with these systems, politicians when emphasizing 'education, education, education' in their rhetoric, should not just mean education for school children, but parents too, especially those parents that are not fully acquainted with the operational aspects of the British system of education.

Mental health issues

It estimated that in the UK, one in four people suffer from mental illnesses (Gilbert 2003). The incidence of these illnesses is thought to be higher for some groups than others and patterns of treatment interventions do vary by ethnicity.

The Department of Health's innovative census of mental health patients undertaken in 2005 suggested that inpatients from the Black Caribbean, Black African and other black groups were more likely by (33–44 per cent) to be detained under the Mental Health Act 1983 compared with the average for all inpatients (Equalities Review 2007:76).

Against this backdrop of higher incidence of mental health issues, black people do not fair well once they have entered the health care system, possibly because of the distortion of cultural norms by racist perceptions inherent in Western thinking (Fernando 2002). However this position is disputed by some on the basis of inconclusive forensic evidence (Sheldon and Macdonald 2009). To compound the situation, mental illnesses are poorly understood; therefore, the consequences of the illness such as stigma and discrimination can sometimes be much more difficult to deal with than the actual illness (Warren 2003).

Stigmatization can have a profound effect on people's social identity and social relationships, and people with mental health problems not only have to manage the symptoms that they experience, but also have to manage societal reactions (Llewellyn *et al.* 2008:293).

There is merit in ensuring that different therapeutic interventions are adopted to support recovery or stabilization among Africans presenting with mental illnesses. Assessments would need to take into account cultural variations in particular the spiritual dimension, because many Africans draw strength from religion and spirituality. With regards to a diagnosis of schizophrenia, for example, Holford (1982) found that compared to other thought patterns, religious values remain intact, thereby providing a helpful social structure from which to create a base to promote recovery. Obomanu (2003) concurs with this view and highlights the importance of religion among Africans and that they prefer to leave problem solving to God rather than take a chance with an often unbelieving therapist.

Practice implications

The discussion on the characteristics of the African population in the UK and some of the social issues highlighted in terms of cultural representation, identity, poverty, educational attainment and mental illness, all require some social services input. Therefore, appropriate leadership and effective management are critical to make sure that changes are planned for, are given serious attention and are implemented. In order to be certain about what works and who does what, production of evidence is necessary. Evidence based practice has become the norm in social care, and support for research is both political and academic for obvious reasons, that of ensuring effectiveness of social care interventions.

Knowledge of what works, for whom, at what cost, in what circumstances, over what time-scale, against which outcome indicators, how and why, should surely be the main preoccupation of training courses for social workers. All other values and ethics considerations, however exciting to debate, are marginal unless such concerns predominate.

Questions of values and ethics should therefore not be divorced from questions of service effectiveness (Sheldon and Macdonald 2009:89).

What works for African families, at what cost and in what circumstances is not fully understood. The shortcoming is that the evidence is not out there, suggesting that the research is yet to be undertaken. This was highlighted recently by Bernard and Gupta (2008:477) in their review of literature on African children and the child protection system and go on to state:

> we have found that there is a paucity of literature and hard data from research on the specificities of African children's experiences to inform the knowledge base. Where literature does exist, the experiences of African children tend to be merged with those of other black and minority ethnic children.

The change that is required towards producing credible evidence needs the attention of service leaders and managers, after all modernizing the public service agenda acknowledges the importance of effective leadership in making things happen. Coulshed and Mullender (2006) remind us that all social workers are managers who regularly use managerial skills in their practitioner roles. As case managers, social workers are working to a managerialist agenda and are, therefore, well placed to identify gaps in research evidence to support their work with African families, they should then ask of their service leaders that the deficit is rectified in the interest of delivering effective service outcomes for African families. From the perspective of an African centred worldview it is likely to be beneficial to undertake the commissioned empirical research from the perspective of the lived experiences of African people. This is important because

> even though a specific system of knowledge or therapy analogous to that within psychiatry cannot be extracted out of the African traditions of medicine, philosophy and religion that have been documented, it is clear that African ways of thinking about mental and psychological matters (in Western terms) are very different from those of the West. In that sense, an African system is there to be discovered and developed.
>
> (Fernando 2002:157)

Leading the research agenda

It is necessary to have in place, leadership that ensures that the right things are done with integrity (Bennis 2000). This is important given the diversity of presenting. The dedication to make the change happen would require that the leader builds and maintains close relationships with staff, who will in turn provide assistance as required (Ruth 2006, Hargreaves and Fink 2006). To make the shift in convincing staff about the need to change and to find ways to produce credible evidence to support social care work with African families, transformational leadership is likely to be beneficial, and probably the best approach. Goodwin (2006) sees this conceptualization as a process that changes and transforms individuals and is concerned with values and standards.

For transformation to happen, clear communication of vision is critical in order to engage the commitment of staff, by helping them to look beyond self-interest (Dubrin 2007). If the evidence is not out there then practitioners need to engage in research and publish interventions that produce the desired outcomes for users of social care services.

To be effective, social care interventions with African families, as with any other group, requires the support of credible research evidence otherwise the identified problems will continue. Transformational leadership can make this happen because at the core of this style is the leader's capacity to empower team members to transcend their own interests (Martin and Henderson 2001). All that said and done, leaders can demonstrate their commitment to this change by making sure those adequate resources are available to undertake the research.

Service user involvement

The historical accounts and research evidence on the characteristics of the African population living in the UK suggest that Africans do want to have a stake in this society and are seeking opportunities to be actively involved as citizens and stakeholders. The term stakeholder is defined as any group or individuals that can affect or is affected by the achievement of any organization (Freeman 1984:217). Implied in this definition is the need to acknowledge the interdependence between the organization and those who depend on the organization for the realization of some of their goals. With regard to social care, stakeholders can be individuals, the community, local and central government and other professional groups who work alongside social work professional groups. By undertaking a stakeholder analysis, it should be possible to identify the different expectations of the various stakeholders and to develop a map to manage the expectations. Using a systems model can also be helpful in identifying the less visible stakeholders such as those providing support services and those who access specific services. The African families as a stakeholder group would need to be placed within the context of all the other stakeholders. It is important to do so because commentators (Bernard and Gupta 2008, Daley 1998) indicate that there has been little specific attention given to this ethnic group to enable service providers to gain understanding of the specific needs of Africans living in the UK.

Stakeholder analysis helps to identify and to give a rating to those who directly and indirectly affect policy and service delivery. In conducting stakeholder analysis, different methods are often used. One of the most direct ways, is to conduct a survey, asking the stakeholders about their needs and demands, how they evaluate and rate the organization and its services as well as asking stakeholders about the additional projects they would suggest. Such an approach would enable African ethnic groups to have a direct input into service planning. Many Africans would have experienced racism and discrimination, making them vulnerable as a group, therefore care is required when surveying this group to ensure that the interviews are conducted in an appropriate and ethical manner. The results of the analysis would give a social services organization direction concerning its positive and negative aspects. This involvement should be aimed at ensuring improved service quality. Service user involvement is in line with social work values of empowerment, social justice and respect for individuals (British Association of Social Workers 2002).

Interdependency and group work

With reference to mental illness, group work could be considered as a therapeutic model because most Africans will have been socialized in cultures that emphasize interdependence, strengthening the ties between the individuals and various groups such as the family and the community (Moghaddam 1998). To be effective, group work models would need to take into account cultural needs and communication patterns in order to avoid mirroring abusive and oppressive structures in society. Where possible, culture specific groups can be set up using a humanistic model of group work that ensures that methods are democratic. If that is not possible, then Manor's (2000) systems approach could be considered. This approach sees group work as a product of personal, interpersonal and social communication structures. In using this framework an individual's background and relationships with other groups in society is recognized as influencing their group work responses. In this case interventions are therefore targeted wider, including individuals as well as family, friendship groups and professionals. Ward (2002) considers group to be a natural, empowering social work method because its success is dependent on the active contribution of every group member. Cultural influences of interdependent self among most Africans renders group work method a potentially useful approach that could be considered alongside other therapies.

Summary

This chapter has provided insights into:

- Africans south of the Sahara and their historical external influences,
- UK based African population and patterns of migration,
- poverty, education and mental health as an area of particular concern,
- the need to take into account African centred cultural representations,
- the need for social service leaders to address the knowledge gap on African family life through commissioned research.

Exercise

1   Think about the knowledge you need to acquire to enhance your understanding of African family life.
2   Create a research question that can inform your research design relevant to an aspect of African family life.
3   Discuss your research question with your peers then undertake a web based literature search, review the literature and share your results with your peers.

2   Social care and policy context

This chapter will:

- discuss social care policy
- examine policy impact on African families living in the UK
- highlight social care practice implications.

Social care policy comes under the umbrella of social policy, which can be interpreted as a deliberate intervention by the state to redistribute resources amongst its citizens in order to achieve the government's welfare objectives (Baldock *et al*. 1999). By achieving welfare objectives through the activities of various institutions created for this purpose, it is thought that success would bind society together (Jones 2002).

Social welfare provision is therefore aimed at ensuring the maintenance of members of a given community in an acceptable state of health and prosperity through statutory programmes or social effort. In industrialized capitalist societies such as the UK, the organization of welfare is complex and multifaceted. Beneficiaries receive welfare support from work, families, friends, voluntary and state organizations (O'Brien and Penna 1998). Post-Second World War, the UK welfare state took shape, having been influenced by the Beveridge Report published in 1942. The emphasis was on state intervention to assist people in meeting social contingencies around housing, health, education, employment and minimum level of income.

> A Welfare State is a state in which organised power is deliberately used … in an effort to modify the play of market forces in at least three directions – first by guaranteeing individuals and families a minimum income irrespective of the market value of their work or property; second, by narrowing the extent of insecurity by enabling individuals and families to meet certain social contingencies (e.g. sickness, old age and unemployment) which lead otherwise to individual and family crisis; and third, by ensuring that all citizens without distinction of status or class are offered the best standard available in relation to a certain agreed range of social services.
>
> (Powell and Hewitt 2002:6)

Successive UK governments with different ideological positions – Labour and Conservative – maintained a comprehensive and universal welfare system while introducing reforms in order to effect some changes and modifications. The historical development of the welfare state, economic imperatives and internalization by the general public about their expectations from the welfare state ensured the survival of collectivism. Among post-war politicians, there was social democratic consensus in support of creating a capitalist environment and activities that would ensure full employment and, as such, this included a comprehensive welfare system. 'The post-war consensus represented a broad agreement between the main political parties about the legitimacy of state direction of the economy and support for state welfare provision' (Ferguson *et al.* 2002:160).

Both the Labour government of 1945–1951 and Conservative government that took over, 1951–1964, remained committed to welfare provision even though the Conservatives' approach was influenced by a different ideological position. However, of particular interest is that there was also consensus between the main political parties in relation to the exclusion of immigrants from benefiting from some of the provision of the welfare state, even though the numbers of those recruited from the Commonwealth to work increased significantly. As colonized subjects, some of immigrants who were encouraged to come and work in the UK had rights of citizenship and settlement. However Williams (1995:139) commented that they were treated as units of labour rather than individuals with welfare needs, and since they were deemed to have come on their own initiative, no special provision (such as low-cost housing or childcare) were made available, suggesting that this was the beginning of the process of state sanctioned social exclusion.

Alcock (2003) highlighted that during this consensual period, immigration from the Commonwealth countries was encouraged in order to offset labour shortage, particularly in low paid jobs in the expanding welfare service. Critics have also noted that the British welfare system was based upon a racialized understanding of the nature of the post-war population that effectively discriminated against immigrants (Ferguson *et al.* 2002, Williams 2001, Lewis *et al.* 2000).

Against this background, Africans coming to the UK from the former British colonies, as with other ethnic minorities, will have arrived into a foreign country with an established democracy and a young welfare state that had been established for the indigenous white population. The seeds of exclusion were sown then and continued into the 1970s and 1980s.

The welfare state was a (white) British achievement, and most of the black people resident in Britain in the sixties and seventies arrived after the establishment of these national welfare services. This invited an assumption by some that Britain's black population had not contributed to the development of the country's welfare services and thus not entitled to use them.

(Alcock 2003:291)

While acknowledging that racism and discrimination against immigrants existed, the majority of Africans who came to the UK during the 1960s and 1970s wanted to improve their prospects through further and higher education or professional training with a view to return to their newly independent countries of origin as discussed in Chapter 1. At the time, they did not see themselves as part of the established labour force. Some among those who sought paid employment did so to support their studies with a view to return to their countries of origin on completion of their courses of study. The institutions that were charged with the responsibility for promoting individual welfare did not see the need to accommodate specific welfare needs of Africans because they were considered to be transient and expected to return home to Africa. Their temporary welfare needs were never given serious consideration and as such individuals of families relied on charitable giving and self-help community activities to meet some of their social welfare needs.

The two main political parties that interchangeably governed the UK since the creation of the welfare state were influenced by their ideological stance in introducing reforms or developing further some aspects of the welfare state. For example, the pro-market, anti-state ideological perspective associated with the Conservative government of the 1970s and 1980s was in part influenced by neo-liberal thinking in relation to limited state intervention to provide public services. Overall, neo-liberals favour competitive market values and competition is considered to be a good thing because it gives power to the consumer. Large state spending is discouraged because of the likelihood of creating a dependency culture (O'Brien and Penna 1998). However, since the economic downturn in 2008, large state spending to rescue the economy will influence debate and future direction of welfare provision as well as changes in ideological thought in response to the national and international environmental imperatives. It is hoped the debates that shape the development of new ideas from a neo-liberalist perspective would ensure that the needs of Africans resident in the UK are not marginalized. In view of this, the summary that follows might change because of the politics of the twenty-first century.

Neo-liberalism summary

- residual welfare model is acceptable,
- rolling back the state by reducing public expenditure,
- privatization of publicly owned services,
- against nanny state and too much regulation,
- welfare dependency produces an underclass,
- market mechanisms can ensure protection for all.

However, when looking back, it seems that in reality, the reforms introduced in the 1980s and 1990s by the previous Conservative governments did not roll back the state, nor control public spending as intended. Instead they retained universal state services, but managed to introduce some reforms through restructuring of the management and operational practices, suggesting a mismatch between ideological perspective and political practice (Powell 2000). Perhaps the political landscape of the day dictated that which could realistically be achieved.

Other ideological influences have also contributed to the debate on welfare provision. For example, social democracy is based on the belief that governments can be used to alter the distribution of resources for economic and social ends. There is an emphasis on tackling inequalities within the capitalist system by working towards fairness and justice. There is an acceptance of collective provision of the main human services that are paid for through taxation, thereby maintaining the viability of the welfare state.

Social democracy summary

- collective provision of welfare as a basis for a good society,
- shared services are a good idea,
- it is right to collectively pay for welfare services,
- social inequalities are to be tackled through social policy,
- redistribution of wealth through taxation,
- moral principles of solidarity and mutual support.

Both neo-liberalism and social democracy have influenced debates on welfare reform and the development of some of the main ideas behind New Labour's Third Way. It can be argued that the welfare state under Conservative or Labour governments never fully addressed issues of social justice in relation to minority groups because policy makers did not put a value on such issues. Collective contribution towards the welfare state by minority groups did not result in their benefiting from the welfare state on par with the rest of the white population. Among some Africans, it is possible that their lack of knowledge about welfare services entitlements compounded the continued state of exclusion from some welfare services. Having come from countries without systems of state organized welfare provision, they would have arrived with the intention of meeting all their welfare needs through economic activity and paid work. The statement of no recourse to public funds that is included in passports at the port of entry would have reinforced the lack of entitlement and, therefore, it is likely that many Africans would never bother to acquaint themselves with the functions of the various institutions servicing the welfare state industry. Their minds will be focused on just trying to find work. The late 1990s saw an energized and rebranded New Labour in which John Smith, Gordon Brown and Tony Blair played a pivotal role. The language of social justice and inclusion and values associated with the creation of policies and action plans to achieve specific welfare objectives were made explicit (Kemshall 2002). The New Labour party won the election on a pragmatic ticket of the Third Way, a label that has come to be closely associated with New Labour and Blair administration, and at the beginning of the New Labour government minority groups, including African groups, started to become much more optimistic about their potential inclusion into mainstream societal activities.

The Third Way

According to Giddens (1998:26) the Third Way refers to a framework of thinking and policy making that seeks to adapt social democracy to a world which has changed fundamentally over the past two or three decades and which seeks to transcend both old style social democracy and neo-liberalism. On the basis of this framework, it would appear that by rejecting both right-wing pro-market approaches and old left support for state ownership of major human services, this was a critique of the ideologies of social democracy and neo-liberalism because of their perceived failure to produce the intended results. Perhaps the timing of the introduction of this framework of thinking was right because the world had moved on and modern societies had become more complex than had been the case during previous decades and, therefore, a new way of thinking and doing things were needed. 'In part, however, it was also a product of a more pragmatic approach to policy making and service delivery, captured by the government slogan "what counts is what works"' (Alcock 2003:11).

For the Third Way, the emphasis is modernization in response to international, national and political pressures. As with previous governments, New Labour emphasized the need to reform the welfare state because it had been assessed as unproductive, inefficient and probably serving the interests of the professional groups as practitioners and managers (Ferguson *et al.* 2002). Overall collective provision is endorsed, but new partnerships between the state and the market are encouraged. The discourse of consensual cooperation and collaboration is part of the repertoire. There is a shift away from the hard tones that emphasize competition. The need to develop a new relationship between the individual and the community is highlighted. Individualism of the 1980s is sidelined in favour of the social and the communal. This new relationship is couched within the principle of paid work to enable all those who are able to work to come off welfare benefits.

According to Williams (2001), paid work is presented as the:

- first responsibility of citizenship,
- route out of dependency into independency,
- solution to poverty,
- point of connection to the wider world,
- role model to offer children,
- glue that binds society together.

This approach to welfare reform focusing principally on paid work would sit comfortably within the mindset of most Africans who came to the UK seeking to improve their prospects through employment opportunities that are thought to exist in the UK. The extent, to which African families would satisfy eligibility criteria for the new range of benefits such as the working families' tax credit, would depend on their immigration status. As indicated earlier, for some Africans, the idea of seeking welfare benefit support from the state would be new and therefore some would not have an understanding of the way in which the welfare systems are operationalized.

The Third Way summary

- mixed economy of welfare, private/public partnerships,
- collective provision and rationalization of limited resources,
- responsibility and obligation,
- welfare pluralism, provision by a variety of sectors,
- surveillance – inspections to keep a check on quality,
- commitment to tackling social exclusion.

What seems to be emerging under New Labour is a welfare system that has been shaped by ideological principles and political influences from the past. It would appear that there is a convergence with some of the Conservative ideas about the welfare state. According to Blakemore and Griggs (2007:56), the British model combines elements of the liberal or residual type of welfare system with remnants of a social democratic approach. The importance of rights and obligations set the scene of what was to come through the Welfare Reform Green Paper in 1998. It stated, at the heart of the modern welfare state will be a new contract between the citizen and government, based on responsibilities (duties) and rights. This has engaged people in talking about rights, citizenship, obligations and responsibilities. Some suggest that these ideas that are stimulating current debates have been influenced by the work of David Ellwood, an American liberal economist writing in the late 1980s (Deacon 2002). Ellwood argued that poverty cannot be alleviated by cash benefits alone and welfare should be organized according to three principles as follows:

- cash assistance should be temporary,
- ensuring that work pays by, for example, supplementing low wages and offering child support so that to work is worthwhile,
- emphasis on welfare being a contract between the government and claimants. For example, the government has responsibilities towards training and childcare support in order to create the opportunity for people to work, and people must work if they can.

It seems therefore that New Labour may have considered the above principles in putting together policy documents that were meant to guide action plans as evidenced in the following narratives:

Obligations – that as citizens, we must balance our rights against our obligations to society. We have the right to welfare but we also have an obligation to take paid work if we can get it; to strive to reach our educational potential; to cooperate with health professionals and to have responsibility to bring up our children as best as we can and instil in them the values that we hold dear.

Reciprocity – we 'take' in times of need and we 'give back' when we can.

Active citizenship – not to be passive but to get involved, give something back, put some effort into benefiting society.

Social responsibility – to think about the consequences of our actions on wider society and the consequences of not acting when we think someone else is not acting irresponsibly.

In summary these notions framed within the concept of duties include those indicated in Table 2.1.

Overall, the above duties are summed up in the following statement: to help individuals and families to realize their full potential and live a dignified life by promoting economic independence through work, by relieving

Table 2.1 A summary of duties

Duty of government	Duty of individual
Provide people with assistance they need to find work	Seek training or work where able to do so
Make work pay	Accept work
Support those unable to work so that they can live a life of security and dignity	Take up the opportunity to be independent if able to do so
Assist parents with the cost of raising their children	Give support, financial or otherwise, to their children and other family members
Regulate effectively so that people can be confident that private pensions and insurance products are secure	Save for contingencies where possible
Relieve poverty in old age where savings are inadequate	Save for retirement where possible
Devise a system that is transparent and open and gets money to those in need	Not defraud the taxpayer

poverty where it cannot be prevented and by building a strong and cohe-
sive society where rights are matched by responsibilities (Welfare Reform
Green Paper 1998). The proposed duties between state and the individual,
if implemented for and by all, would probably enable most Africans,
particularly those new to the UK, to feel part of the larger community.
Education and training, finding paid work and supporting extended family
members are common aspirations among Africans, and in some cases
normal expectations within most African communities. Therefore, government policies designed to support individuals to receive training geared
towards securing paid employment are likely to be well received, because
Africans who migrate to the UK are prepared to, and do want to, work.
This is demonstrated by their acceptance of low paid positions well below
their academic qualifications as encapsulated within the following
quotation.

> Generally, respondents were fairly well educated. As a result, many
> had experienced de-skilling and downward social mobility on entering
> the British labour market. One half of all the workers interviewed had
> attended primary or secondary school, and 49% had acquired tertiary
> level qualifications. Of the latter, half held vocational or professional
> qualifications and half had academic qualifications.
>
> (Evans *et al.* 2005:11)

Among the social welfare changes that are under way, some are more
prominent than others subject to resource availability. In relation to social
care, the trend towards privatization of social care borrowed from the previous Conservative government has continued under New Labour suggesting that the mixed economy of welfare remains.

Partnership working with the voluntary sector continues to be encouraged. Regulation and tougher controls are in place. The introduction of
mandatory NVQ (National Vocational Qualifications) for those working
in the social care sector has forced employers in that industry to ensure
that staff receive relevant training. The social care sector does employ a
significant number of Africans, particularly women, who are therefore
included among those that should be afforded training. Before mandatory
NVQs were introduced, it is likely that African social care workers would
have been excluded from partaking in training. While the changes are wel-
comed by some, critics highlight limitations in that the principle of a needs
led service remains aspirational, and instead social care is currently a
resource led service even though the current administration has put more
money into social care than the previous one. 'New Labour has substan-
tially increased the total amount of government expenditure on social services and social care though this area remains – in relation to social
security, health education, and many other areas of government spending –
the Cinderella service' (Blakemore and Griggs 2007:241).

To benefit from direct or indirect state social care provision, the issue of social rights to social care as citizens can expose some of the complexities of entitlement. Some African families find themselves excluded from some social care services as non-citizens due to their immigration status or unfamiliarity with the UK benefit system. A study of low paid employment among migrants in London found that only 16 per cent claimed any kind of state benefit (Evans *et al.* 2005). In situations where individuals approach social services for help, unfortunately it is the frontline social care practitioners who find themselves in positions of having to explain to potential service users unacquainted with UK welfare systems that their claimants to welfare support do not meet government policy criteria due to their immigration status. For some Africans, the exclusion can lead to isolation, feelings of not belonging and, in some cases, this exclusion leads to the development of African specific community groups for support and self-help. Such developments create exclusive and separate social care provision at a time when national cohesion is being thought of as a positive way forward. The development of separate social care provision exclusive to specific African community groups would not be unique because research evidence indicates that others have travelled a similar path.

> Some of the problems have led black groups in the country to develop separate welfare services, designed to meet the needs to which public welfare services cannot, or will not, respond. Separate provision can be found in the voluntary and community sectors, where large numbers of black and ethnic minority organisations serving distinct ethnic communities and particular service needs.
>
> (Alcock 2003:192)

It can be argued that separate welfare provision is not desirable because it reinforces the divisions between black and white people who might continue to see themselves as them and us – citizens and non-citizens. Because of these concerns, it is necessary to explore the ideas about citizenship in some detail since rights of citizenship are affected by inequalities in provision of social care as well as other welfare state services.

Citizenship

Within the Third Way model, citizenship plays a part in terms of entitlement to welfare benefits. There are links between citizenship, immigration status and entitlement to welfare services. The discussions on citizenships and the welfare state have been influenced to greater or lesser extent by the works produced by Marshall (1950). He considered citizenship to be the set of social relations between people and the wider society of which they are a part. Marshall argued that citizenship forms the basis for engagement with the institutions of society, while these institutions, in turn, promote the circumstances in which the exercise of citizenship is possible. From this line of thought, citizenship and social welfare would be seen as mutually integrative.

It seems that Marshall's view of citizenship places too much reliance on the state as the basis of social citizenship rights. There is no reference to the erosion of citizenship through powers exercised by the state through its officials and professional staff. For example, immigration officials, health and social care practitioners carry out duties on behalf of the state in such a way that creates barriers to engagement with these institutions of society. Additionally there is no recognition of social divisions based on race, ethnicity and culture (Blakemore and Griggs 2007). Citizenship can also be used as a means of excluding people from rights – for example, the debate on asylum seekers. Social divisions based on race needs recognition because citizenship as rights based discourse is embedded in the nation state and identity, therefore citizenship can be a component of identity, linked to a sense of belonging and having rights. The links between citizenship and identity were evidenced by the results of the Oldham study.

In their research on citizenship, ethnicity and identity after the Oldham riots, Hussain and Bagguley (2005) found different citizenship identities operating in the same community. Some of the different citizenship identities are highlighted in Table 2.2.

Overall, citizenship identities of the older generation were considered to be weak because their experience of migration made them feel insecure, as visitors who might return to, or be sent back to, their countries of origin. But the younger generation born in the UK were found to be confident about their sense of belonging, their country of birth, with equal rights as British citizens and having the right to be different within Britain. This is echoed by Brah (1993:26), in which she asserts that African Caribbean and Asian young women in Britain seem to be constructing diasporic identities that simultaneously assert a sense of belonging to the locality in which they have grown up, as well as proclaiming a 'difference' that references the specificity of the historical experience of being 'black' or 'Asian' or 'Muslim'. These constructions of diasporic and hybridized identities would suggest that intergenerational uniformity and commonality that would normally be expected to occur were not apparent. In the Oldham study, the researchers concluded that:

> When people make statements about British citizenship they are expressing quite fundamental ideas about where they belong, about

Table 2.2 Identities

First generation	Subsequent generations
Naturalized born elsewhere	Ascribed natural right by birth
Resident in foreign country	Secure in belonging in Britain
Insecurity linked to migration	Hybridized identity

who they are and what rights they have. In this context these rights entail duties and obligations from the state and others towards them as British citizens.

(Hussain and Bagguley 2005:421)

The findings of the Oldham research about the 2001 riots on citizenship ethnicity and identity have relevance to other minority groups with similar experiences of migration such as Africans living in the UK. Their lived experiences are likely to determine how they see themselves and that self-assessment would probably fit into the following four categories:

category (1) new arrivals – work permit holders or asylum seekers,
category (2) settled and naturalized,
category (3) citizens by birth to naturalized parents,
category (4) born in UK to new arrivals retaining similar status to their parents.

For individuals in each category, they are likely to think about their identity and citizenship in different ways based on place of birth, migration pattern and lived experience. It is highly likely that those that fall within categories (1) and (4) will see themselves as visitors in a foreign country. Those who fall into category (2), some might feel settled and a sense of belonging, but others might feel insecure because of their naturalization status and for the fact that they would have been born elsewhere. Young adults born to naturalized parents, in category (3), are likely to feel confident about their British identity and African ethnicity. Being alert to the variety of identities can enable those needing to engage with African families to look for appropriate ways to connect with such families. By allowing space for a conversation that allows families opportunities to articulate how they see themselves in relation to the rest of the UK population can support meaningful engagement.

However, in some cases, racism based oppression can sometimes contribute towards judgements about entitlement to welfare benefits for some Africans. In times of economic recession, for example, the experience of the past eighteen months, the situation can be particularly difficult because of suspicion that black African people do not belong in this country and therefore can be excluded from accessing welfare services delivered within the framework of the welfare state.

The exclusion of black service users from welfare provision in Britain is not, however, just a product of racist discrimination fuelled by suspicion of illegal immigration; at a more general ideological level it runs deeper than that. The development of services within the 'welfare state' of the post-war era was very much a product of the national (and nationalist) politics of the time (Alcock 2003:291).

UNIVERSITY OF WINCHESTER
LIBRARY

Media stimulated nationalist politics tend to be pronounced during periods of economic downturn, adding to the suspicion that all black Africans are non-citizens and benefit scroungers. It seems to be important that misrepresentations of citizenship and identity are counteracted with credible evidence about the exclusion of this group from accessing welfare benefits and the net economic contribution of individual Africans to the local economy. As with other minority migrant communities, they do not just take, as perceived by some, but make a contribution to the national gross domestic product. For example, it is estimated that in 1999/2000 migrants in the UK contributed £31.2 billion in taxes and consumed £28.8 billion in benefits and state services, a net fiscal contribution of approximately £2.5 billion (Gott and Johnston 2002:iii).

While accepting the idea that the state can intervene and assist people in meeting essential welfare needs, this is conditional upon satisfying stipulated criteria and these criteria can sometimes have a disproportionately adverse impact on those that are recent migrants to the UK, such as those from Africa south of the Sahara who may not pass the citizen rights test. This exclusion would suggest that those Africans migrating away from poverty in their countries of origin are likely to find themselves at the bottom of the poverty ladder and not entitled to welfare benefits. The extent of poverty among some African families can lead to many more social problems. As agents of the state, what can social services departments do to alleviate poverty related problems within African communities? Because African families are affected by government social care policies, subject to their legal citizen status, can social workers make a difference in minimizing some of the problems arising from poverty? Opportunities to secure paid employment would be part of the answer.

Overall, the answer ought to be yes, because social care is the provision of individual support to those in need and are unable to provide such support for themselves. Families that are likely to need social care support would come within category (1) – new arrival into the UK – whose numbers have increased since 2007. It is reported that the increase in this category of the African population, brings correlating poverty related social problems with significant negative impact on the children in these African communities (AFRUCA 2008).

Traditionally, social care support is sometimes provided by other members of society on a voluntary basis and, at times, by paid social care workers (Alcock 2003). Voluntary social care support is common practice within African communities and this voluntary activity could benefit from direct social work input because, according to Horner (2002:10), the task of the social worker is to facilitate the resolution of social problems and conflicts at the personal level. It is different but not separate from social care, which is looking after individuals on behalf of the community. The engagement of social worker with individuals in need means that they will have insights into the impact of poverty on African family life in the UK. Therefore, social work as a professional activity that oversees the delivery of social care support could use the limited clout it has to meet some of the needs, as appropriate, to ameliorate social problems within some African communities.

The operation of social work and the provision of social care are based upon processes of identifying the needs of individuals and providing services in response to these (Alcock 2003:98).

Social work's clout comes from its identity as a profession that has the essential characteristics associated with most professions in which individuals belonging to a professional group are prepared to exercise their skill in the interest of others. In this case, the focus is specifically on African families.

According to Finlay (2000), these professional characteristics that can be put to good use for the benefit of others include:

- altruism → members act in the best interest of their clients,
- trustworthiness → giving impartial, expert and confidential advice,
- skills → members have specialist skills,
- knowledge → professions have a body of theoretical/scientific knowledge,
- control of entry → professions determine eligibility,
- competence → specified training and assessed standard of competence,
- code of conduct → written codes of ethical conduct to be adhered to,
- organization → self-regulate and monitor standards,
- autonomy → professionals can make independent judgements and decisions,
- power → professional influence public policy,
- professional culture → codes of conduct inform acceptable behaviour.

The list above would suggest that a professional group, so identified, such as social work, would have shared values guiding their practice. A value can be recognized as an enduring belief that a specific mode of conduct is personally or socially preferable to an opposite mode of conduct (Roakeach 1973:5). Values determine what is considered to be important and worth striving for, and therefore give rise to general standards and ideals by which we judge our own and others' conduct; they also give rise to specific obligations. The specific obligations for social workers are derived from the professional core values suggesting that social work is expected to promote respect for human dignity and pursue social justice through services to humanity, integrity and competence (British Association of Social Workers 2002:2).

From this list of professional characteristics, there are two that warrant specific attention, namely, skills and knowledge. Social work training equips practitioners with essential skills and relevant knowledge specific to the practice of social work. Drawing on their knowledge and skills and supported by credible research evidence of the effectiveness of social work interventions, social workers can confidently identify the nature of support that can be made available to African families experiencing social problems. Social workers can also rely on research evidence about the most effective approaches that could be used when working with community groups as partners in the delivery of social care within the membership of a given community.

Sheldon and Macdonald (2009:67) confirm that the evidence of social work's effectiveness is today of increased volume, based on robustly designed studies.

An evidence based body of knowledge about UK citizenship and eligibility to social welfare, and clarity about who can have recourse to public services, would enable practitioners to be clear about that which is possible to achieve in terms of positive changes, while highlighting the likely consequences of the gaps in social care provision for African families.

Skills and knowledge can also assist social workers in working with dilemmas they encounter, for example the paradoxical position of social work. It is a profession that has traditionally identified itself with those who are oppressed or marginalized in society, and yet it is sustained and funded by the same society – welfare state dependent. Policing certain socially agreed norms, and at times resorting to the law to compel compliance, does not sit comfortably with the idea of working in partnership with those who use social care services (Beckett and Maynard 2005). What seems to be important is that practitioners acknowledge that care and control dilemmas will continue to exercise them and that control used appropriately is not the opposite to care, provided that statutory powers are not abused to meet professionals' needs, to allay their fears of losing control. Lack of knowledge about specific needs of African families categorized by their immigration status and citizenship can engender fears of losing control. Such fears may lead to inappropriate care related decisions being made. I would argue that managers and leaders of social care services have an obligation to support front line staff through ongoing professional development and through creating appropriate environments for the conduct of effective anti-oppressive social care practice. This important role for managers and leaders of social care will be considered further in the next chapter by examining some of the organizational and leadership literature based evidence and the application of that evidence to modern social care enterprises.

Summary

This chapter has provided insights into:

- political ideologies that influence state welfare provision,
- citizenship and conditions for welfare entitlement,

- the role of social care practitioners in implementing welfare policies,
- the exclusion of some groups from utilizing the welfare state,
- partnership working with African communities.

Exercise

1 Identify ideological differences between neo-liberalism and the Third Way.
2 How do these differences inform social care policies?
3 What is the relationship between citizenship and individual rights to social welfare?

3 Organizational and leadership context

This chapter will:

- discuss the organizational context of social care provision,
- examine current thinking on leadership and management,
- suggest ways in which leaders can influence appropriate service delivery to diverse African communities.

Organizations are entities created for a stated purpose. They are created on the basis that more can be achieved by people working in harmony and towards a stated purpose than by individuals working alone. As such, the organization as a concept provides categories for sorting, organizing and storing experiences. Organizations pervade all aspects of life: social, economic, political, cultural, religious, communal and family (Hatch 2006, Pettinger 2000). Social care is delivered by individuals who belong to a variety of organizations of different sizes, configured in a variety of ways. These organizations include voluntary, private and statutory agencies. The current government agenda has forced statutory social care service leaders to engage with the existing literature on leadership and management to assist them with formulating ways of working by creating organizations that are likely to support staff to give of their best and to produce desired outcomes.

It is also claimed that organizations, such as those expected or required to deliver social care services, arise from activities that individuals cannot perform by themselves or that cannot be performed as efficiently and effectively alone as they can with the organized effort of a group (Hatch 2006). As with most organizations, social care organizations have identifiable structures. Organizational structure refers to the relationships among the parts of an organization as a whole and these structures can be physical or social as highlighted below:

- physical structure → is associated with buildings and geographical location,
- social structure → is associated with units, people, their roles and work groups.

Physical structures are self-explanatory in terms of building designs and layout where people are housed for work purposes, the objects within buildings and agreed décor. However, further discussion on physical structures can be found below.

Social structures

In relation to social structures of work organization, the human factors are significant in terms of the way in which the work is distributed, the clarity of roles and distinctive units of work. Within these distinctive units there will be formal systems of rules, tasks and authority relationships which control how people are to cooperate and use available resources. The design of the formal structures reflects how managers utilize the various components of the organization towards goal attainment. Because the structure is associated with the allocation of formal responsibilities and division of labour, it is argued that organizational structures provide employees with a settled and orderly working life (Martin and Henderson 2001). To that end organizations are designed and structured in order to (Pettinger 2000):

- ensure effectiveness and efficiency,
- divide and allocate work,
- clarify responsibility and authority,
- establish patterns of management and supervision,
- establish means by which work is to be controlled.

The distinctive variations in the components of the organization structure are affected by the nature of the work, the technology used, the expertise of staff, the stability or volatility of business environment (Burns and Stalker 1961).

Physical structure

The ideas about physical structures of work organizations have been influenced, in part, by Elton Mayo's Hawthorne studies conducted over a period of five years during the late 1920s and early 1930s focusing on productivity and the physical environment in which delegated tasks were carried out. The results of his research showed that by changing the physical structure, creating a separate space that allowed group interaction away from the surveillance of their supervisors, there was noticeable behavioural change. The group members' interaction had a positive effect on performance, highlighting the importance of groups in affecting the behaviour of individuals at work. From those results, he was able to make deductions about what managers ought to do and that the task of management is to organize spontaneous cooperation among employees. This task remains evident in present day social care management of teams and group working.

Overall the conclusions from the research were (Pugh and Hickson 1996):

- people are motivated to work by social needs,
- they satisfy their needs through social relationships at work,
- the work group exerts more influence on a worker than do the incentives and controls used by management,
- supervisors are effective only to the extent that they can satisfy those they supervise.

The evidence based conclusions from the Hawthorne experiments have relevance to social care organizations as echoed by experienced practitioners working within social care enterprises.

> People have a natural propensity to associate with one another and they care what 'their' group thinks about them. To be motivated, they need a management style that maintains and builds on this spontaneous cooperation in groups, takes a genuine interest in both the individual and the group, provides new interest from time to time and also recognises that workers, employed in an enterprise which has been artificially created to achieve certain ends, do think about what good their work is to the wider society. All this makes perfect sense in social work.
>
> (Coulshed and Mullender 2006:38)

While the focus was initially on the physical structure, the initial research theme took a back seat when compared against the value placed on human interaction labelled the Hawthorne effect. The human relations approach based on the Hawthorne studies has had an impact on management theory and practice, because it offered an alternative to Taylorism – scientific management that paid specific attention to efficiency and left a legacy that continues to influence management thoughts processes in relation to the discourse of output measures, functional analysis of performance and performance indicators (Coulshed and Mullender 2006). Apart from challenging the scientific management theory and its one best way of undertaking specific jobs, the human relations approach has also been credited with influencing much of the thinking about the importance of adequate communication systems across organizations. However, critics of the human relations approach highlight some concerns about overgeneralizations (Pugh and Hickson 1996, Handy 1993). The extent to which the human relations approach might have influenced open plan physical layout of statutory social care working spaces in the twentieth century is an issue for debate. However, up and down the country, practitioners are no longer shut away in individual office spaces and, instead, they access computers through a 'hot desk' arrangement in large open spaces and have easy access to colleagues and managers enabling practitioners to share concerns and to get immediate support when dealing with difficult and complex cases. However, the downside of working in open plan layout is that there could be constant interruptions that can detract individuals away from specific lines of thought in relation to planning social care interventions.

The ideas about social structures are associated with the division of labour within work organizations. Weber's ideal bureaucracy is one way that has continued to influence the thinking about distribution of responsibilities and assignment of work tasks within organizations (Hatch 2006). During the 1960s, research on organizational social structures, considered environments and their likely effect on structure (Lawrence and Lorsch 1967, Burns and Stalker 1961). The results of their empirical studies produced the approach that became contingency theory. The focus of the research was on the impact of different environmental conditions on the structures of work organizations. The research was informed by the thinking that there was no one right way of structuring work organizations. From this research, they concluded that the structure required for any given organization is contingent upon conditions or the complexities and changes to the environment. Contingency theory therefore, suggests that an organization will be successful if it consciously adapts its structure and its administrative arrangements to the tasks that need to be done. The contingency argument suggests that in stable environments, mechanistic organizations perform well, but in rapidly changing environments, the organic organization will do well. For the purpose of this discussion, the environment is conceptualized as:

> an entity that lies outside the boundaries of the organization. It influences organizational outcomes by imposing constraints and demanding adaptation as the price of survival. The organization, for its part, faces uncertainty about what the environment demands while it experiences dependence on the multiple and various elements that comprise its environment. It is this interdependence and uncertainty that explain organizational structures and action in the environment conceived by modernist organizational theorists.
>
> (Hatch 2006:63)

Based on their empirical work, Burns and Stalker (1961) identified two management systems, mechanistic and organic structures, that lie on two ends of a continuum defined by the stability and instability of the environment in which the organization operates its business. They highlighted a number of characteristics for each system (see Table 3.1).

In summary, mechanistic organizations are characterized by complexity, formalization and centralization.

Table 3.1 Characteristics of management systems

Characteristics	
Mechanistic structures	Organic structures
Hierarchical arrangements	Horizontal network of authority
Defined roles and responsibilities	Low formalization
Centralized decisions	Decentralization of decisions
Written rules and procedures	Mutual adjustment
Close supervision with authority	Prestige linked to expertise
Vertical communication	Lateral communication

Source: adapted from Hatch 2006:111.

Organic organizations are characterized by simplicity, informality and decentralization.

However, it is important to note that for most organizations, they are likely to fall somewhere towards the middle of the continuum, particularly in large organizations with subsystems that interrelate to make the whole organization. With the idea of an organization as a system, a working definition has been put forward as follows:

> a thing with interrelated parts. Each part conceived as affecting the others and each depends upon the whole. The idea of interrelated parts emphasises that, while all systems can be analytically broken down for the purpose of scientific study, their essence can only be identified when the system is confronted as a whole. This is because subsystems interdependence produces features and characteristics that are unique to the system as a whole.
>
> (Hatch 1997:35)

Social care organizations can be viewed as systems made up of complex subsystems such as finance, information, people and the service and they all interrelate to make the whole. These social care organizations are open systems that take in inputs from their environments. The inputs are then transformed to become outputs and the outputs can be assessed in relation to desired outcome.

In giving further consideration to social care organizations as systems that interact with their environment, it is possible to assess the environment in which such organizations operate, then analyse the operational structures to determine fitness for purpose. If not, this calls for change towards a perfect fit. Social care organizations possess a mixture of characteristics reflecting the complex formal nature of social care arrangements that require some centralized decisions on one hand and the need for flexibility and informality on the other at front line level so as to relate effectively to individual needs of service users. In addition to environmental influences, mechanistic and organic social care organizations operate within and are influenced by cultures that have been developed over time and therefore the concept of culture needs further discussion.

Culture

To support an analysis about fitness for purpose, the ideas relating to organizational culture can have a part to play because there is a link between organizational structures and cultures. According to Handy (1993), culture conveys the feeling of a pervasive way of life, or a set of norms. Within work organizations this culture represents a deep set of beliefs about the way work should be organized, the way authority should be exercised and how people are rewarded and controlled.

Schein (2004:17) defines the culture of a group as a pattern of shared basic assumptions that are learned by a group as it solved its problems of external adaptation and internal integration, that has worked well enough to be considered valid and, therefore, to be taught to new members as the correct way to perceive, think and feel in relation to those problems. The elements upon which cultural sharing is based include artefacts and linguistic symbols. Lawler and Bilson (2010) suggest that the meaning of culture within work organizations is established through socialization to a variety of identity groups that converge in the work place. These interpretations suggest the need to have some understanding of organizational culture given the relationships that exist between culture and structure and their impact on human behaviour within work organizations.

An understanding of organizational culture in relation to social care organizations is useful because culture influences behaviour among organization members through shared meaning. So, generally, the purpose of culture is to provide members with a sense of organizational identity and to generate commitment to the core values. If the culture is a healthy one, members can contribute to the effectiveness, efficiency and service quality. If the culture is unhealthy, it is likely that values based destructive conflict will ensue. This type of affective conflict can result from poor interpersonal relationships leading to inadequate group performance. However, issue based substantive conflict between organizational members is beneficial as it can stimulate debate and discussion and lead to better decision making (Rahim 2002). In social care, it is therefore important to develop organizational culture that fosters substantive conflict while managing affective conflict so as to minimize performance deficits.

Hugman (1998) seemed to think that affective conflict as a result of the clashes of values and principles could be contributing towards the decisions made by some practitioners to opt out of the social work profession. It would be important therefore that managers put in place systems that help to minimize destructive affective conflict. In highlighting his concerns about the changing nature of work and organizations Charles Handy provides a framework that can be used to analyse organizational culture, while acknowledging the limitations of such a framework in view of the ever changing nature of employment patterns and the way people choose work in the twenty-first century.

Drawing on the characteristics listed in Table 3.2, social care organizations can be viewed as having a role culture that determines how things are done through the use of procedures and rules informed by statutes. This culture conforms to Weber's (1947) ideal type bureaucracy and Burns and Stalker's (1961) mechanistic structure. Task culture is also apparent in the sense that social care practitioners work in teams, control how they work and must work creatively in response to individual service users' needs. This culture is associated with an organic structure that draws resources from all parts of the system. A mixture of cultures influences organizational design and, as such, person and power cultures have had limited influence on the design of social care organizations because these organizations do not have one 'boss' at the centre of the web with the power to make most major decisions. Additionally, social care organizations are not subordinate to the individual as would be the case in a person culture type of organization.

Given the dominance of the bureaucratic mechanistic nature of statutory social care organizations, while operating in a fast changing turbulent environment, it is likely that these organizations will encounter difficulties when attempting to meet stakeholders' demands. Some of these stakeholders will be African families with specific needs that are less familiar to some managers, leaders and front line practitioners. For positive changes to take effect there is a need to ensure that issues of diversity informed the working structures and cultures of social care organizations. Within these structures and cultures, supervision of practitioners will have an important part to play and managers, through supervision, can provide support and exercise control to ensure that inclusive positive changes are implemented. Therefore leadership and management would be expected to play a significant role in directing the change in line with current thinking on managerialism and modernization to ensure that those who use social care service are

Table 3.2 Types of organizational culture

Type	Characteristics
Power	Web-form, centralized power, few rules, political, risk taking
Role	Procedures, rules, regulations, position power, inflexibility, predictability, temple-form
Task	Net-form, teams, adaptability, creativity, control of own work, speed, judgement by results
Person	Cluster-form, shared influence, expert powerbase, mutuality, organization subordinate to the individual

Source: Handy 1993, based on Harrison 1972.

fully involved as active participants in their care. Such an inclusive approach if implemented would benefit African families.

> Managerialism is a discourse which sets out the necessity of change; a set of tools to drive up performance; and means through which an organization can transform itself to deliver a modernized notion of public purpose to a modern conception of 'the people'.
>
> (Newman 2000:58)

For the change to happen, managers will need to get the work done through the people they are responsible for. Literature on what management is refer to the ideas documented during the 1920s by a French mining engineer, Henri Fayol, who summarized the lessons of his own experience into a number of General Principles of Management. It is indicated that he drew attention to the importance of management in the government of undertakings; of all undertakings, large or small, industrial, commercial, political, religious or any other (Pugh and Hickson 1996:97). The undertakings were packaged into six groups to include: technical, commercial, financial, security, accounting and managerial activities. Fayol argued that these essential functions could be found in most senior jobs. Perhaps twenty-first century social care senior jobs are no exception and the most significant among these activities is management. From the analysis of industrial undertakings emerged his definition of management highlighting the universal aspects common to most organizations.

His definition of management (Fayol 1949, cited in Pugh and Hickson 1996) included five elements stating that to manage is to:

- forecast and plan → looking to the future and drawing action plans,
- organize → material and human,
- command → maintaining activity among staff,
- coordinate → harmonizing activity and effort,
- control → ensuring conformity with established rules.

In this definition and the clarification of a group of six activities present in most management jobs as well as the formulation of fourteen principles that informed his practice, Fayol managed to influence the direction of future management research. The fourteen principles covered many of the ideas in current literature on management. Examples from the list include: division of work, authority and discipline; units of command, direction and subordination; order equity and stability; initiative, motivation and communication. He is the earliest known proponent of a theoretical analysis of managerial activity – an analysis which has withstood a half-century of critical discussion (Pugh and Hickson 1996:101). Given that the five elements have provided a system of concepts with which managers may clarify their thinking about what it is they have to do, and that many who write on the subject of management have been influenced by this theoretical analysis of managerial activity, it would seem appropriate that social care managers give some consideration to this way of thinking about what they do and why they do it in that way. More importantly, managers could make use of current social care research evidence in assisting the adaptation of the original ideas to make them relevant to the ever changing demands of modern social care organizations that must respond appropriately to the specific individual needs within diverse communities. For example, planning for statutory social care with children and families within a given planning cycle requires that managers have accurate and up to date information on African families in their catchment area as potential users of statutory social care services to enable them to accurately predict courses of action.

In relation to an exploration of what managers do, Mintzberg (1973), focused his research on work activity and noted the fragmentary nature of a manager's job. From these observations he deduced ten managerial roles, grouped into three distinctive areas as follows:

- interpersonal role → as figureheads, as leaders and a liaison person,
- informational role → monitoring, dissemination and spokesperson,
- decisional role → entrepreneur, disturbance handler, resource allocator and negotiator.

These ten roles provide a useful starting position from which social care managers may reflect on what they do within their job role. Mintzberg highlights the informational role as central because it interrelates with the other two in support of management activity. Lack of accurate information on African family life is thought to have had an effect on some child protection decisions (Chand 2008). This suggests that managers could use their interpersonal role to acquire essential information that can then inform the decisions to be taken. What is emphasized is that management is an art and that managers should try and learn continuously about their own situation and the configuration of their particular organization. Another important area that continues to receive considerable attention in relation to the modernization agenda set by the present Labour government is the importance of effective leadership. Social care organizations remain in the spotlight due to well publicized cases of tragedy that are subsequently investigated such as the deaths of baby Peter and that of Victoria Climbie (Laming 2009, 2003). Social care managers are expected to promote joint up working and ensure that the sharing of information between agencies does happen as part of safeguarding children. As well as giving attention to ideas about effective management of social care organizations, it is important to also consider leadership.

Leadership

Leadership and management are bed 'buddies' but different. Having considered above what management is and the roles performed by managers, the next section deals with leadership and leaders. As part of the changing nature of social care, there is an emphasis on the need to understand service users' experience of care. The market principles of the 1980s continue to influence current thinking. It is also expected that there will be further changes towards a more equal relationship between social care provider and user of social care services than has been in the past. This transformation implies a move away from the notions of passive recipient to an active user of services choosing from social care options (Martin and Henderson 2001). In return, the users of social care services are expected to take a keen interest and to become more responsible for their well-being than previously, in line with the current thinking on rights and responsibility and active citizenship, hence the emphasis on appropriate leadership because things cannot carry on as before and in the old ways.

However lack of insider knowledge, vulnerability and fear may cause dissonance between provider and user of services. Therefore, this changing nature of social care demands a particular type of leadership. The Scottish Leadership Foundation (2005) took the position that leadership is necessary at all levels of organizations and that effective organizations need to nourish both competent management and skilled leadership at all levels. The importance of visible leadership across the whole organization wherever social care services are delivered and the articulation of the vision of the organization, as well as explanation of how the organization will fulfil its vision, was acknowledged as a helpful starting point towards change. For those at the top of the 'tree' and occupying leadership positions, the message was that they must provide effective models for the rest of the organization. The combination of empowering, enabling leadership and effective management are likely to create successful social enterprises (Scottish Leadership Foundation 2005). To get to a position of clarity about appropriate leadership within twenty-first century social care organizations, it would be beneficial to consider some ideas from existing literature on leadership.

Traditionally leadership has been studied within the context of management focusing on personal characteristics of effective leaders. According to Ruth (2006), leaders are people who are influential in other people's lives. Such individuals are likely to possess characteristics such as being inspiring, approachable, supportive with clarity of vision. Influential leaders are able to think clearly about the other person and what that person needs. In this case, people have to be thought about as individuals as well as collectively. Additionally, effective leaders think about what is happening in the wider context, having a vision of how things could be different: this being a key feature of effective leadership. These ideas sit well within the field of social care, suggesting that these ideas are embedded in the everyday reality among social care practitioners who must be approachable, supportive and positive and maintain a clear vision of what they need to achieve with each intervention. In theory Africans who approach social services for support ought not to experience poor service if this way of working is part of everyday reality.

Goodwin (2006) considers vision to be the essence of leadership because it provides a positive image of what a service could become by following an identifiable path. Leaders with a vision are able to hold out a view of the picture that can excite and inspire other people. Therefore an effective leader is one who acts as a facilitator, team builder, enabler, thinker and developer of other people (Ruth 2006). Most publications on leadership give some attention to theories of leadership to stimulate debate about the direction of future research on the subject. Since the notion of leadership in social care has steadily been emerging on to the research agenda, some attention to the documented theories on leadership would be a useful thing to do. Traits, style, contingency and transformational leadership theories are included in this section in order to show the journey travelled thus far with hope that future practitioners might choose to investigate further applicability or otherwise of these theories to twenty-first century social care leadership.

Traits theory

This theory assumes that leaders are in possession of special qualities that make them stand out. The emphasis is on the importance of the leader rather than the situation in which the leader would be operating. Traits theory is based on the 1920s research about in-born superiority (inherited traits). However, no universal characteristics could be identified among those who were born into leadership roles. It was also realized that the personal qualities and attributes of those in leadership positions were also shared by a wider, diverse group of people who were not in leadership positions.

Because of these reservations, no serious further research has been undertaken since then but the debate continues. According to Lawler and Bilson (2010:39) leadership might have become considerably sophisticated in many respects, but there is still a strong feeling in some camps that it is innate qualities of an individual, rather than any qualities or skills that have been learned or developed over time, that suit them for leadership. So the notion of born leaders is still around.

Style theory

Research conducted after the Second World War produced style theory with a focus on the behaviour of leaders. The research highlighted that task oriented behaviour facilitates achievement of objectives, while relationship behaviour helps followers to feel good about themselves and their situation. Some of the well known investigators on the subject include Adair (2002) and Blake and Mouton (1964). From their research Blake and Mouton developed a grid which rated a leader's actions according to task orientation and people orientation. Adair adopted a functional approach to leadership and at the core of the process are interrelated tasks with the aim of achieving a common task. He added that a good leader is someone who can ensure that the needs of both the individual and the group are met at all times.

Contingency theory

The 1970s research on leadership suggested that different situations demand different kinds of relationship and that the leader's effectiveness depends on how well their style fits the context. Contingency theory shifted the emphasis of leadership research from person-to-person to person-to-context with an emphasis that leaders ought to adapt their leadership style to accommodate the changing circumstances. The extent to which leadership styles could be changed to suit the context and situation, and the leader retains their effectiveness, is questionable.

Transformational theory

Research carried out during the 1980s focused on the ideas about transforming individuals by winning hearts and minds, offering vision, sense of purpose and direction. Transformational leadership is a process in which the leader engages with potential followers as individual people. The connection ultimately becomes moral in that it raises the level of human conduct and ethical aspiration of both leader and followers and thus it has a transforming effect on both (Goodwin 2006:38). Perhaps the essence of transformational leadership is that leaders transform the way their staff members see themselves and the organization, suggesting that the core of this style is the leader's capacity to empower team members to transcend their own interests and, through collective involvement and participation, take ownership of the organization's vision (Martin and Henderson 2001).

As with most subjects, organizational leadership continue to exercise the minds of those who have an interest in the subject matter. Theories as systems of ideas can assist with the study in order to deepen knowledge and understanding, particularly knowledge that has practical application. Theories can also assist with the analysis of complicated situations such as those arising daily within the field of social care. From the process of analysis it may be possible to discover effective means of dealing with complicated scenarios. Unfortunately many leadership theories exist, but do not always fit neatly together, and there are many disagreements among theorists. However, highlighting the disagreements would indicate engagement and an understanding of the specific subject. One of the main criticisms of the existing leadership theories is that they are based on research that did not include in the various studies the views of marginalized groups such as African people. Based on her study of leadership traditions in the history of black women in America, Parker (2005:92) suggests that twenty-first century theorizing on leadership should reflect the interplay and struggle of the multiple discourses that characterize post-industrial society. She expresses a view that African American women's strength as leaders have gone unacknowledged, devalued and otherwise marginalized, and encourages future investigators to take an inclusive approach that recognizes diversity. This view is supported by Parks (2001:118) and states: 'the responsibility that Black women traditionally hold in the family suggests that the family is a traditional locus of Black female power which demands a particular leadership style'. Rather than a traditional leader, what Antonio Gramsci calls an organic leader who assumes power through heredity, wealth, or military might, black mothers are organic leaders who naturally emerge to facilitate group survival and gain power through responsibility and history. There are similarities between the experiences of black mothers in the United States of America and the experiences of African women in the UK. Ellis (1978) found that African mothers in the UK have to cope with very severe pressures because they take on the role of breadwinner, student and mother. These responsibilities demand a particular leadership style that is yet to be researched. Survey participants indicated that same pressures experienced by African mothers in the 1970s are still evident today. Other suggestions for inclusion in future research is couched under the umbrella of bicultural strength that helps black leaders operating in a predominantly white organization to function effectively (Davidson 1997). Finding out how such leaders straddle the two worlds – one at work (white) and one at home (black) – would add new knowledge to the existing literature on leadership that takes into account diversity issues.

Diversity management and leadership

In relation to social care with African families living in the UK, a great deal could be achieved through an inclusive approach. Working for and with diversity in organizations is an argument which has assumed the same status as working with and for democracy in broader society. It is a perceived force for the good and has robust personal, social, economic moral and ethical rationales which are difficult to refute (Maringe *et al.* 2007). Diversity management and leadership within social care organizations require that the existing organizational structures and cultures are evaluated and adapted to ensure fitness for purpose. Making adaptations ought not to cause too much strife among practitioners because of the nature of their work and their commitment to anti-oppressive practice. The definition of international social work suggests that social workers are expected to protect and care for those citizens deemed to be in need of protection. Implicit within the aspects of protection and care is that social workers are fully conversant with the nature of diversity, of need among all those citizens in need and that social workers are starting from a position of valuing diversity. Valuing diversity starts from the position that people's differences as users of social care services or workers are an asset rather than a burden to be tolerated.

> Organisations or departments established specifically to deliver social work or related services may be thought to have a special responsibility to consider issues of gender, ethnicity, culture and religion, age, disability and health, class, poverty and issues affecting gay and lesbian people, since these are now recognised as essential considerations in the delivery of social work itself at the practitioner/service user level.
>
> (Coulshed and Mullender 2006:219)

Acceptance of this special responsibility by organizations or departments and taking appropriate action will benefit all those who use social care services including African families because front practitioners will know that these considerations are an essential requirement of their job. The changes required in terms of additional demands to ensure appropriateness of service delivery to all, makes it imperative that front line practitioners receive development support to enable them to improve their performance. The improved performance will be achieved when there are changes in attitude and behaviour in the way social care is delivered, for example to African children in the care system. This development requires reappraising one's values and reorientation and using feedback to help and heighten awareness about the impact of practitioner behaviour on others.

As well as responsibility for developing others, leaders and managers in social care have a responsibility for monitoring and evaluating effectiveness. With monitoring, the attention is on checking out progress against service objectives (Cameron 1990). This provides a focus on the specific issues and knowing when they have been achieved; for example, the recruitment of a specific number of foster parents representing the population profile served by a given local authority.

Objectives are helpful if they are clearly stated, explicit and measurable. In social care practice, objectives assist in answering the question – how shall we know, over and above subjective feelings, that something worthwhile has happened? Evaluating performance involves checking out components of outcomes against set objectives and baseline measures taken. In this regard, being clear about the measures that would best represent improvement is important. Social care practitioners should know how to continuously evaluate their work. To demonstrate improved performance in a given area of activity, it is necessary to have a combination of quantitative and qualitative measures of performance. Quantitative measures are more likely to be robust and convincing to stakeholders, but qualitative measures are equally important. Increasingly within the public sector, managers have to operate within significant constraints: they have to operate with probity, within policies and procedures that are intended to protect the interests of a wider constituency – the service as a whole, its employees, its clients and the general population (Flynn 1997). Because of the wider implications, public sector leaders and managers must be accountable for the four Es, namely, effectiveness, efficiency, economy and equity. These variables continue to dominate the measurement of performance in public services.

Effectiveness

In general, effectiveness is about making progress towards the outcomes desired by particular stakeholders. Cameron (1990) suggests four approaches that can be used to evaluate organizational effectiveness:

- goal accomplishment
- securing needed resources
- healthy internal processes
- satisfying strategic constituencies.

In considering goal attainment, social care enterprises or individuals would be judged by how effectively they attain pre-determined goals or how close their outputs come to meeting their goals. Securing needed resources is linked to finances and healthy internal processes which relate to trust, cooperation and minimal conflict. Satisfying the interests of many constituencies or stakeholders is equally important. Therefore, effectiveness considers the extent to which the various demands are balanced and met.

Brechin *et al.* (2000) refers to effectiveness as the extent to which an activity or programme achieves its intended objectives. At times the measurement of the level of effectiveness is through examining the nature and severity of unwanted side effects.

Efficiency

This is a measure of the use of resources: it is the ratio between the results gained from the use of specific resources. It takes into account the outputs achieved for given inputs. An efficient activity produces the maximum output for any given set of resources inputs. Sometimes output measures used to assess efficiency are raw activity measurements such as numbers of visits, or episodes of care that may not build up to effective service overall.

It is therefore necessary to demonstrate that the inputs are used well in producing outputs. This is the basis of many performance measures expressed in terms of cost of a service per unit of service delivered. Politicians often emphasize the view that public sector workers must implement efficiency measures and do more with less financial inputs.

Economy

This means being thrifty, working within available resources, not wasting anything and spending money carefully. Staying within budget tends to be the main focus. It does not necessarily relate to whether money has been spent on the right thing. Being accountable for money is important in public services and sophisticated systems have been developed to handle complicated financial data (Martin and Henderson 2001). Budget reporting and the budget cycle have become dominant factors in measuring performance. According to Flynn (1997), a manager who can demonstrate that the services were effective, the service users were delighted and other stakeholders were satisfied will not last long if the budget is consistently overspent. So delivering an effective service efficiently and economically should be the desired outcome.

Equity

The emphasis is on fairness in terms of availability of services for a given population. The creation of the internal market for public services was intended to increase the range and choice of services, so that different services could be provided for different people. Unfortunately, the desired outcomes have not been achieved. Instead, the internal market created inequitable services as highlighted through the 1997 White Paper and its reassertion of fair access to services in relation to people's needs, irrespective of geography, class, ethnicity, age or sex. It signalled the need for performance measures to assess equity in the provision of services.

Using the four Es framework as basis for measuring organizational performance can help leaders and managers to demonstrate how well the organization is doing in relation to services provided and delivered to African families particularly in those areas where success is apparent and the results can be communicated in a transparent manner. Sharing success is important because it makes those who carry out the work feel good and sustains motivation to continue to do better. In taking into account the classical approach to leadership, social care leaders are accountable and responsible for all aspects of the work of the organization as demonstrated in high profile cases within social care in which the person at the top of the 'tree' is suspended pending results of an inquiry, resigns or is dismissed. Therefore the approach remains relevant and can be a basis for directing operational activities.

Summary

This chapter has discussed:

- organizational context of social care,
- the concepts of structure and culture,
- the importance of management and leadership,
- the relevance of monitoring and evaluating services.

Exercises

1   In thinking about specific social care needs of African families, how can the management of diversity ideas be used to ensure that the provision of social care services from different providers fills an existing gap in take up?
2   What structural and cultural organizational changes would need to be implemented by statutory agencies to ensure that their procedures and practices do not discriminate unfairly against African families?

4   Student survey

This chapter will:

- present survey results,
- provide brief comments about the main themes that emerged.

Although the heading for this chapter is 'student survey', the convenient sample included existing, and former students who had attended the University of Reading but were now qualified practitioners undertaking front line social work. Having taught and/or teaching the participants, and had the opportunity to listen to some of their experiences, there was an expectation that this sample group would provide useful information drawn from their lived experience in Africa and the UK. It is recognized that the information obtained from this group is specific to members of this group; however, some common experiences emerging from this group were also noted from other studies on African family life. Comprehensive studies on this subject have not been carried out within African countries possibly due to limited financial resources or lack of interest in the subject matter. In the UK, this has not happened either, possibly because of the methods used to determine priorities for funding empirical studies, and yet various academic papers (Chand 2008, Graham 2007, Barn and Harman 2006, Boushel 2000), all point to the shortage of empirical evidence on African family life. My interaction with students on health and social work undergraduate and postgraduate programmes over a number of years suggested that students needed to learn and understand African family life because they were unsure whether the knowledge gap was real or imagined. The uneasiness made some students think that they might find it difficult to meaningfully engage with African families in their professional capacity. It is hoped that the views expressed by this group of survey participants could make a contribution towards putting the issues raised on the research agenda by generating interest among potential researchers and funders. The emphasis on evidence based practice highlights the need to generate empirical evidence to inform practice interventions with African families.

Research process

During 2008, forty survey questionnaires were circulated to all African former and existing social work students at the University of Reading who are currently living in the UK, the majority of whom are mature adult women learners and are also parents of school age children attending local schools. However, at 20 per cent representation, mature male participants within this convenient sample group were above the national representation in the social care sector in the UK and in most African countries. The social care sector remains dominated by women internationally. A significant male representation is an anomaly, possibly due to limited opportunities in other professional programmes which traditionally attract male applicants. Thirty-four out of forty questionnaires were returned and it was evident that participants had given serious thought to their comprehensive answers to the questions as there were no omissions or blank spaces. A response rate of 80 per cent is very good for a postal questionnaire based survey. Out of the six non-respondents, two questionnaires were returned to sender because the addressees had moved to new and unknown addresses.

Results

Role of religion, faith and spirituality

All respondents concurred on the significance of the role of religion and spirituality among Africans. It was more or less stated as the norm, the done thing for most people. The participants' subjective experiences within their communities appeared to have informed their specific statements in response to the question. They relied on what they knew and had experienced first hand. They indicated that religion and attendance at places of worship enabled individuals to connect with like minded African people that engendered a sense of belonging. The church provided opportunities for people to meet and develop friendships as well as providing safety in numbers at congregations. Most of the participants thought that a significant number of Africans who had a religious faith were active Christians and that their active participation gave them hope and ways of sustaining resilience to overcome some of the negative complexities of the Western lifestyle. Reference was made to life threatening illness and the role of religion in helping individuals to come to terms with known medical conditions such as HIV and AIDS. The practising of religion was also seen as closely linked to issues of identity because those people who come together for worship and common prayer engender solidarity and cultural identity that enable individuals to feel a sense of belonging and self-worth. Religion was reported to be important because it informed lifestyle choices in terms of doing 'good' by others. Overall the responses were very positive about the role of religion, faith and spirituality. However, it was acknowledged that regular attendance at church was not always possible for some families because of the types of jobs they were engaged in and in some cases attendance reduced after people had been living in the UK for a long time. This decline in church attendance after a number of years of residence in the UK might suggest aculturization because church attendance for the majority white population continues to decline compared to earlier periods during the nineteenth and twentieth centuries.

Examples of statements in response to the question on the role of religion include:

- integral part of life and religion gives hope and paves the way for trust,
- fundamental source of guidance,
- provides a coping mechanism against a hostile environment,
- spirituality is a tool for liberation,
- promotes and sustains emotional well-being,
- provide motivation to remain positive about life,
- tool for healing against the pain of racism and oppression,
- promotes valuable spiritual health by nourishing the soul.

The estimation was that 75 per cent of all Africans living in the UK consider themselves to be religious and the majority of these Africans regularly attend places of worship as Christians or Muslims. Obomanu (2003) concurs with views expressed by these participants and the idea about leaving problem solving to God is well established within African communities because it is believed that God will provide solutions to their problems. Ridge *et al.* (2008) found similar results in their study in that many African individuals turned to religion to help them cope with difficult and at times traumatic life circumstances including illness, uncertain immigration status and poverty. Perhaps the majority white population might have believed similarly two centuries ago at a time when there was significant material poverty.

Mortality, death and final resting place

Based on the evidence submitted, older African people deal with mortality and death in a way that is common to most people in that they would want to die in dignity and not to burden the living. However there was a consensus on avoidance of loneliness in old age and that most older people would want to be laid to rest in their countries of origin. In some African communities, members club together to raise the necessary funds to meet the costs of repatriation. Repatriation of the deceased is considered to be important so that they can join the spirits of the departed ancestors. Some people select to return when they know that their illness is terminal in order to be certain that appropriate funeral rights would be carried out.

Prior to repatriation, there is usually an extended period of mourning when community members visit the home of the deceased to offer condolences and pay homage as a sign of respect to the deceased. The majority of the respondents thought it was a duty to attend and to support the bereaved family and minimize isolation. Representative statements in answer to the question on mortality and death include:

- death is sacred and many would want to be buried in Africa,
- ceremonies are conducted according to the traditions of the country of origin,
- some make pre-paid arrangements,
- support from the church community is particularly helpful,
- deceased will be a lost soul if buried in a foreign land,
- maintain African practice if buried in UK,
- would not want to die in a nursing home,
- respect for the dead is important.

It was acknowledged by all that it was likely that poverty will force some people to rethink their burial plans as African communities become smaller due to tighter immigration controls. It was also noted that for some Africans who had lived in the UK for most of their adult life, they may select not to be repatriated to their countries of origin. When that happens the wishes of the family are respected and a combination of religious and traditional African burial practices is observed.

Dual culture

Participants indicated that this was a difficult area for many African parents because they wished their children to have a better life than they had, hence the reason for migration, and yet they also valued their African culture and traditions. Communication was singled out by all participants as the key ingredient to enable parents and other family members to share the essentials of African family life, highlighting similarities and differences, so that young people will be equipped with the tools to select the 'good' from each culture. It was thought that by involving young people in organized community and church activities outside school would support the families' efforts in transmitting African values. The difficulties arising from dual cultural experiences were considered to be particularly acute among young people who had experienced school life in Africa prior to migration. It was indicated that for many of these young Africans, settling into the British education systems, making new friends while conforming to African cultural norms within the family were aspects singled out as potentially damaging and sources of ongoing tensions within families. The emphasis was that parents continue to look for ways to prevent tensions and potentially damaging conflict as well as finding methods that they can employ to deal with problems when they arise. Church based communities were reported to be working tirelessly to support families in preventing problems from arising and/or during periods of conflict. Overall, the methods and techniques used by families to support their children in balancing bicultural demands were varied as illustrated below:

• explaining contradictions between cultures,
• education via oral tradition,
• use of mother tongue and involve children in food preparation,
• take the children on holidays to countries of origin,
• allow the young people to mix and match that which works for them,
• acknowledging and appreciating difference,
• attendance at cultural festivals,
• parental role modelling,
• make accessible bicultural literature.

The responses to the question on biculturalism demonstrated an appreciation that culture is not static and that parents have a responsibility to enable the young people to deal successfully with the changes they face. The changes would be part of a new culture that could be labelled an African/UK hybrid. This hybrid culture has implications for identity. Perhaps the African young people can decide on the interpretation of this new culture as they experience it.

Child discipline

Reference to religious values and the law featured prominently among the responses as the main guides to how parents exercised discipline within the family. Talking and explaining the consequences of bad behaviour were highlighted as particularly important. Discipline was not seen as the preserve of just the immediate family. Friends and the church community played a part in reinforcing parental wishes. The idea that in Africa it takes a village to raise a child appears to have been transported to the UK, hence the reference to friends and the church community. Other methods stated were similar to practices in most families such as setting clear boundaries, rewarding good behaviour and withholding privileges such as pocket money for bad behaviour. Four participants stated that on some occasions they had used or witnessed physical punishment such as pinching and smacking even though they were aware that it was against the law. A summary of the methods used by African parents to discipline children include:

• tough love and sharing hard facts about the consequences of indiscipline,
• set and maintain clear boundaries,
• mean what you say no pretence,

- telling off,
- smacking,
- grounding,
- remaining firm and resolute,
- help with chores in the home,
- give praise and reward good behaviour,
- continue to explain expected behaviour,
- work with church leaders to reinforce family values,
- threaten to send the children back home to Africa.

Like most parents, Africans do expect their children to be well behaved and do try very hard to instil discipline using a variety of methods. However, lack of extended family support as would be the case in their African countries of origin while working unsocial hours does create additional pressures for some African families resulting in discipline breakdown. Concerns were expressed that external influences on children can make it difficult for parents to discipline their children in ways that they know to be effective, leaving parents and children in confused states. It is an area that was thought to need attention in terms of supporting parents and children who are going through transition and at the same time wanting to make a success of their life in the UK. Some participants thought that African parents are perceived as harsh when it comes to disciplining their children. Fears about potential allegations of child abuse have made some parents become uneasy and tend to act cautiously instead of being spontaneous.

Child rearing practices

Communal upbringing and respect for all adults were noted by all participants. These aspects influenced most of the practices in relation to how children would be expected to conduct themselves among their peers and in the presence of adults. Boys and girls are expected to take on different responsibilities in adulthood, therefore their upbringing reflected that. For girls, they are expected to contribute and learn to become responsible for all the housework as well as looking after children in their adult life. In view of this girls are taught how to do domestic work such as cooking, washing and cleaning. Boys are expected to provide for the family therefore must achieve good grades at school to pave the way for a successful career in adulthood so that they will be able to take care of their family. However, it was acknowledged that these gender specific practices are changing, be it slowly.

Examples of specific responses to the question on child rearing practices include:

- breast feeding is an expected norm,
- during the period of nursing, babies and toddlers are carried on the back in a sling – usually by females,

- babies sleep in the same room with parents and sometimes in the same bed,
- older children mainly girls look after little ones,
- good conduct in public is an essential requirement,
- good behaviour and manners are expected at all times and more so in front of visitors,
- children are every adult's responsibility,
- a child belongs to the whole community,
- children are taught to share and individualism is discouraged,
- children are expected to undertake age and gender specific chores,
- kinship care is a fairly common practice,
- honour and obey mum and dad and become responsible for their welfare in old age,
- adults are not addressed by their name – but uncle or aunt,
- praying before meals and bedtime is common practice among African Christians.

There was an acknowledgement among most of the participants that variations exist between countries and between regions within countries and that practices change with time due in part to the degree of external international influences. Living in the UK meant that families are making some adjustments as a way of coping with new environments. However, in their view, most known successful African families are thought to have achieved their successes without ditching their cultural heritage. As such, these families were seen as role models on issues of child rearing practices.

Marriage practices

The consensus was that marriage was valued by most Africans and that the groom's family expects to provide stipulated resources to the bride's family. This exchange of goods and/or money is standard practice although variations are emerging and critics of bride-price arrangements see it as an out of date practice because it interferes with the balance of power between couples. Marriage is conducted between the couple in the presence of a large extended family. A point that was highlighted by many of the participants was that marriage practice was an exchange of relations between families who can then establish and secure useful alliances. It is like two clans coming together through the institution of marriage and hopefully look after each other's interests. Strong views were expressed in favour and against the bride-price and such strong views and debates are also taking place across the African continent south of the Sahara, suggesting that incremental change away from the payment of bride-price is likely to be achieved when the majority of women join forces to challenge some of the negative aspects associated with this aspect of marriage practice because it is the women who appear to be disproportionately affected in a way that makes their husbands the dominant partners in marriage. The diversity of views expressed by survey participants include:

- bride-price is the norm and perceived as a natural requirement in all Africa countries south of the Sahara,
- men feel superior and dominate women because of this payment,
- women are made to feel like the property of men,
- bride-price gives men rights over children of the union,
- sustains women's subordinate position and lower status,
- perpetuates unfair power imbalance in marriage,
- men assume excessive authority over women,
- makes it easier for men to leave their wives,
- respect is lavished on those who pay bride-price,
- bride-price strengthens the relationships between two families,
- payment is a token of respect and appreciation to the in-laws,
- for some women bride-price provides a perceived sense of being truly married.

The statements as listed above suggest that bride-price payment has an impact on African men and women in different ways. Because it is such a common practice, change towards its abolition may still be a long way away. It was indicated by some of the participants that Africans living in the UK conform to this practice. In cases of interracial marriages between a UK male national and an African woman, payment of bride-price is still expected to be paid and many do.

Main pressures experienced by families

Participants highlighted that most Africans see formal educational qualifications as their main ticket towards securing well paid jobs, and to achieve this end result the families put enormous pressure on themselves to succeed academically. The balance between parental study and paid work to support the family as well as being there for the children to support and encourage them to achieve good grades is an issue that was echoed by all. They commented that for many families there was constant juggling that went on relentlessly. For some parents, their overseas student status makes it very difficult to raise the necessary tuition fees through paid work while at the same time trying to give appropriate attention to their course work. It was also indicated that some African children experience racism and discrimination within the school system resulting in under achievement. It was noted that some parents who may have had very high hopes for their children become disillusioned with the British education system to the extent that they send their children back to their African countries of origin to attend senior school as boarders returning to the UK for short periods during school holidays. Another area of concern involves young people who attend school in the UK while their parents work as permit holders. When these young people complete their secondary education, they cannot progress into higher education under home student arrangements, but can only do so as overseas students. For most of these African students they will be unable to raise the tuition fees causing real hardships and disquiet within families because back home in Africa, the extended family members make assumptions that there will be a natural progression into higher education for all who manage to secure residency in the UK. Poverty, prohibitive tuition fees and racism were considered by participants to contribute significantly to the pressures experienced by African families. These pressures were thought to be contributing to mental health problems.

On the issue of employment, the main concerns centred around lack of opportunities for well paid jobs, lack of recognition for non-British qualifications, poor promotion prospects and having to constantly prove oneself to white colleagues and senior managers. Stereotypes about what Africans are like and are capable of doing within work environments caused frustration, anger and despondence. Immigration status affected employment opportunities compounding poverty because individuals who fall within this (in limbo) category do not have recourse to public funds. It was stated that some survive on clandestine patterns of employment. As with all families, childcare remains a big problem. For African families, the situation can be compounded by isolation, being away from the support of the extended family and not having adequate resources to pay for good quality childcare and yet parents have to work to meet basic needs. All these pressures affect the well-being of family members leading to a breakdown in relationships. Divorce among Africans living the UK was estimated to be rising, but hard evidence is not available. Participants' estimates were based on divorced people they know within their communities. The changes to family composition due to divorce are likely to affect employment chances for women, in particular if they have small children, thereby adding to existing pressures.

Additional information

In an attempt to offer participants the opportunity to add further information, the last question was included as a catch-all. However, it yielded some interesting comments and suggestions as well as re-enforcing previously stated positions. The main points raised are as follows:

- it is normal for Africans to offer food to guests and to refuse would offend, and guests included those visiting in a professional capacity,
- direct eye contact is not the norm, it is learnt behaviour on arrival in UK and people need to be allowed time to adjust,
- deferred gratification can result in parents sacrificing good accommodation for the family and this tends to have a negative impact in children and home learning environment,

- private fostering remains a reality among some Africans,
- family breakdown and unreported domestic violence is a big problem,
- discipline and parental control should not be seen as abuse,
- for newly arrived Africans, they need to know that race is an important aspect for looked after children within the care system and this needs to be addressed if successful outcomes are to be achieved,
- there are distinct hierarchies that are observed within most African families,
- there are tribal divisions that are reflected in language and religious practices,
- families are important to most Africans and older people are respected by the whole clan,
- families are constantly grappling with a variety of unfamiliar systems and most important of all are home and school life,
- acknowledging that most Africans experience racism and as such they need genuine support from those who care – not those who fake.

These points are a mixture of expectations, practices and difficulties that form part of everyday experiences among some African families. Improvements can result from external support and from within family units when the family figures out the best ways to make the most of the opportunities that exist in their adopted country. External support could come from social services working alongside community groups to carry out preventative work.

Summary

The results of a questionnaire survey of existing and former Africans students studying social work at the University of Reading have been presented. Participants drew on their observations and lived experience in Africa and the UK to provide some insights into some of the issues of importance to them and their communities. Participants highlighted how these issues affect the lives of many Africans as they negotiate their way and adapt to living in the UK. These results form the basis of discussions in the remainder of the chapters.

Exercise

1   Select from the results issues raised that suggest strengths of African families.
2   Consider how these strengths could inform social care interventions with African families.
3   Identify the issues raised that should be of concern to social care practitioners.
4   Reflect on how you might deal with these issues within your practitioner role.

5 Social, cultural and economic pressures

This chapter will:

- discuss economic, social and cultural pressures,
- critically examine life transitions,
- highlight implications for social care policy and practice.

Employment

Pressures in relation to employment are significant because most Africans as highlighted in Chapter 1 migrated to the UK in search of a better life through education and employment. However the reality can be different to the image that they had before arriving in this country. The following quotation sums up the views expressed by most of the participants referred to in Chapter 4.

> Employment by some measure is the most harrowing. One has to deal with issues such as discrimination, trying to fit into a new culture that is different from what one is used to, expectations and performance benchmarks can be different when compared to your white counterparts. Behaviour and sometimes interpersonal relationships can be hard to establish and to predict what sort of interpretation and label that will be put to it. Sometimes, one feels alienated or sidelined when certain decisions are made. Some colleagues can be less tolerant and this often creates mistrust and further alienation.
>
> (Practising social worker: participant (19))

In addition to the above, the most harrowing aspects that were stated include the lack of recognition of African qualifications leading to poor employment prospects.

As a result, a significant number of African migrants accept poorly paid jobs. And even then, the indication is that they still have to constantly prove themselves to management that they can carry out simple tasks. This suggests that some employers consider Africans to be less able. Racism was stated to be a problem because of its impact on the individual's self-confidence, but this came as no surprise that racism still existed in this century. Another area of concern that impacted on employment opportunities as seen through the eyes of this group is associated with immigration status with particular reference to asylum seekers. Not being allowed to work causes people to become very depressed and lose all hope for a better future; the very reason for coming to the UK. It was noted also that some self-funding African students find themselves in a dilemma because of the limited time allowed to work, whilst international fees remain high. For some it becomes a case of work to pay the fees or attend class, do the assignments, then worry about the fees at a later stage, knowing very well that being a debtor to the university means no graduation.

The pressures associated with unemployment and underemployment among Africans as articulated by these participants are confirmed by other studies (Equalities Review 2007, Evans *et al.* 2005, Daley 1998, Alcock 1997).

The employment related pressures generated feelings that are evident in the following quotation:

> Based on my experience of working with African families; the following have been the main pressures – loneliness, isolation, frustration, not feeling respected, hopelessness, depression, not being heard, not trusting, feeling constantly judged, self doubt and always having to prove oneself.
>
> (Practising social worker: participant (21))

It is likely that an accumulation of employment related pressures can affect family life and in some cases result in family breakdown or mental health issues.

What is significant, and probably not fully appreciated by those external to the African community is the relentless pressure exerted from abroad in their countries of origin to meet the expectations for financial support from their relatives in Africa. It is a cultural norm that has yet to change. The evidence to suggest that this pressure is unlikely to ease in the near future is based on the state of play with regard to remittances to Africa. For example, the money Africans sent abroad to their families in 2006 was estimated at US$20 billion (Moyo 2010). The level of material poverty affecting the lives of so many people in Africa makes it difficult to ignore. Most Africans find themselves just caving in, and do what they can to help, even though their own situations were less favourable than they had hoped prior to their arrival in the UK. This suggests a conflict between African values of communal support and interdependency approaches to living arrangements and the values of independence and individualism prevalent in the wider community. It is becoming more pressing for Africans to manage the conflict for health reasons and for their emotional well-being to minimize family breakdowns. The interdependency is turning to dependency, because the Africans living in the UK appear to receive virtually nothing in return. Traditionally, this is not how it was meant to be, because the emphasis was on reciprocity. This pressure is not unique to Africans living and working in the UK, because evidence shows that those in paid employment in African cities and towns experience similar demands for financial support (Apt 2002, Harden 1992). But those living in the UK do have to deal with a distinct additional factor of being black and living in a predominantly white country where some individuals still retain racist attitudes and would like to see all black people return to Africa. Survey participants were clear about their experience of racism and discrimination confirming what is already known based on empirical evidence.

Education

The responses about the pressures associated with education included themes relating to the experiences of adults in further and higher education as well as children in schools as illustrated by the following quotations:

> Almost all Africans consider education as a means to enhance employment prospects, while at the same time balancing full time education and full time work is indeed trying. Sometimes the choice of what you are studying makes it even harder to guarantee employment prospect and this can add considerable pressure on the family and most will end up doing menial jobs, far below their potentials since there are mouths to feed and other family members to support back home.
>
> (Student participant (7))

'There are expectations from family members back home to be highly qualified because in Africa, higher education is synonymous with better opportunities' (student participant (11)). 'High academic achievement is ranked very high in Anglo-African families and societies, therefore children and young people are often pressurised to study hard, go to the best schools and try and get the best jobs' (student participant (16)). 'This is bad. Our children are ignored in class because they are black and if they under perform, there is no one to help. No one cares' (student participant (6)).

These statements from four respondents were selected because they represented the views of the majority – thirty participants. In considering college and higher education there was unanimous agreement that opportunities do exist, but at a price. Among students who are not eligible for UK home fees, they struggle in an attempt to balance three things: paid work + full time study + normal family life. The indication seems to suggest that they end up doing all three badly.

Racism and discrimination were cited by all respondents as something they had experienced or witnessed and think that they and their children can achieve much more and lead better lives if their opportunities were not diminished by racism and discrimination. Embarking on a social work career gave each participant a window of opportunity for doing good by others, learn to effectively challenge oppressive systems and to achieve personal goals. It was noted that the pressures associated with experiences of racism and discrimination are common to many people from other minority ethnic communities and many academic books have been produced about the extent and manifestations of race discrimination, and legislation to tackle the problem is in place. Formal investigations and inquiries have been conducted with a view to find workable ways to deal with the problem by recommending lists of action points, but the problem is proving to be a hard nut to crack. More recently the Equalities Review (2007) confirmed the extent of progress achieved while highlighting outstanding deficits to achieving desired outcomes. Perhaps the Africans can play a part in contributing to the action plan alongside others who wish to see real change away from oppression to liberation. As well as their meaningful engagement in challenging racism induced oppression, Africans living in the UK can be supported and encouraged to reflect on their life as they make the transition towards biculturalism as they embrace the UK way of life. The next section deals with the ideas for consideration around transition.

Transition

Including the survey participants, Africans who decide to migrate and settle in the UK for a variety of reasons, would need to embrace change with all the complexities of transition that lie ahead. Experiencing a transition involves undergoing a process of change within the life course, demanding personal growth and role adjustment.

(Crawford and Walker 2003)

To adapt and make a successful transition, migrants need support to enable the learning and internalization of the new culture in terms of how life is conducted in the UK. For individuals in transition, it would mean a challenge to the existing beliefs informed by core values from the country of origin. Individuals are likely to be expected to adopt new roles within their new home in the UK and society at large. For some, the adaptation can be a mental and physical struggle. However, the migration based change can also involve positive growth. The growth aspect can enable newcomers to the new environment to achieve their goals, in terms of the aspects of their lives in Africa which spurred them to progress and to migrate. On arrival as black African migrants, identity issues are likely to arise for adults and children as they straddle between two cultures.

Erickson's (1965) lifecycle theory could be useful in terms of analysing transition development stages. He predicts a crucial development task people undergo is that of identity versus role confusion. The thinking behind this prediction is that successful resolution of this emotional conflict supports individuals with a strong self-concept, enabling them to move on to the next development stage. The argument is that unsuccessful resolution leaves the person confused or selecting to adopt the opposite identity to that which would be expected, producing an unhealthy outlook.

Erickson's (1965) constitution of life development has relevance and merit; however, for migrant adults and children, the order of experience would be different because identity formation is closely linked to adolescence, limiting applicability, particularly, in the case of adults, suggesting the need to draw on other theoretical propositions of life tasks.

Accepting the theoretical propositions of life tasks as multi-directional, plastic and imbedded in personal history can be beneficial (Baltes 1987). Such theories can enhance understanding towards the development of a positive identity. Therefore, ideas about enhancing cultural acculturation can be used. This acculturation can be supported by improving status, language use and personal contact with welcoming people, and ongoing personal cognitive appraisals (Berry 1995).

One of the major difficulties for most African migrants is the loss of social networks in terms of family, community clan and friends. These networks would normally support individuals in a variety of ways including solving personal problems. Linking new arrivals with established African communities including the church could enable the recreation of new support networks. Most African cultures are collectivist; therefore interdependence is a valued norm, thus individuals would not feel out of place within the context of shared group identity. The UK societal and cultural norms are likely to present many challenges for the newcomer, therefore enabling them to understand the environmental context in which the transition is taking place is important.

African families need time to adapt and adopt the UK lifestyles and expectations (student participant (10)).

Bronfenbrenner's (1979) ecological model could also be considered here. The emphasis is on isolating interrelating structures that support individual development and growth.

These structures could include:

- micro system → family and peers within the church,
- exosystem → local community, health and social care organizations,
- macro system → wider cultural and political structures.

Depending on individual circumstances, it is possible to use this model as a tool to support interventions decisions. The interventions would aim to involve the different structures within the context of culturally appropriate set-ups. Africans new to the UK need support by clearly explaining the workings of the various interrelated functional social systems. A clear explanation of the various interrelated functional social systems is important, because to a newcomer, they can be a complete nightmare. Social care practitioners should not underestimate the importance of this activity. From this it can be expected that fully supported Africans will find it easier to make a success of their transition. Supporting individuals through transition can also draw on ideas of attachment. Attachment theory suggests that through life individuals use strong attachment figures as safe bases from which to explore their surroundings (Crawford and Walker 2003).

Exploration of attachments for individuals prior to leaving their countries of origin can help African migrants to move on and explore their new environment. Chamberlayne *et al.* (2000) suggest that biographical histories and past narratives, in line with current needs, should be considered when offering support to individuals going through transition. Narratives would be particularly beneficial to Africans because most of them come from communities with established oral traditions and are therefore likely to share their histories with a sensitive, non-judgemental and supportive professional practitioner.

Most Africans who migrate to the UK do so in order improve their life chances through education and employment. However some will not secure jobs of their expectation, resulting in disappointment that can lead to stress and poor health.

These changes in relation to occupation and finances are part of significant life transitions and tend to have a domino effect (Holmes and Rahe 1967). This domino effect challenges Erickson's (1965) sequential stages theory which suggest that individuals face one transition at a time. It would seem therefore, Rapoport and Rapoport's (1975) triple helix model acknowledges this complexity whereby transitions in family, occupation and status are intertwined and co-dependent. Recognizing this interaction among those who care would ensure that planned interventions are holistic. Another aspect that needs to be taken into account is that often, expectations about life in the UK tend to be based on the publicity through the media, thus unintentionally promoting unrealistic expectations. Hopes can be dashed, leaving people alienated. Those whose job it is to care can do more to minimize the difficulties associated with major personal change. Africans on arrival in the UK will encounter difficulties due to the adjustments they have to make socially, culturally and psychologically. Use of stage models of life transitions have a part to play, but there are limitations when working alongside migrants from different cultural backgrounds. However, drawing on theories accounting for sociological and multi-directional factors could complement stage models with a view to produce effective interventions, while acknowledging that these models have been developed with a particular culture in mind; therefore, such theories and models may need to be adapted to make them relevant to those in transition and are between cultures. In addition to transition theoretical propositions and models that could be considered when working with and supporting individuals from Africa, ideas relating to liberation could also have a part to play. The next section addresses the concept of liberation.

Liberation

Participant (21) cited feelings that are associated with internalized oppression. It seems therefore appropriate to discuss ways in which helpers can work with Africans experiencing hopelessness and self-doubt towards liberation, given the common currency of empowerment prevalent within the helping professions.

Andersen and Hill-Collins (1998:50), state that the experience of oppressed people is that the living of one's life is confined and shaped by forces and barriers which are not accidental or occasional and hence avoidable, but are systematically related to each in such a way as to catch one between and among them and restrict or penalize motion in any direction. It is the experience of being caged in: all avenues, in every direction, are blocked or booby trapped.

The description above relating to the experience of oppression echoes some of the feelings expressed by survey participants suggesting a sense of being caged in and desperately looking for ways to be liberated from the trap. The narratives seem to suggest that they were subscribing to a view that internalized oppression causes people to feel bad about themselves and other members of their group. These bad feelings are associated with low self-esteem. This low self-esteem can be contradicted by holding out an alternative perspective that reminds people of their true nature and worth (Ruth 2006). It is incumbent on the social care practitioner to find ways to give people hope and to continually look for ways to help oppressed people to use life affirming expressions (Saleebey 2002).

Liberation techniques have been suggested at two levels, personal and leader. For this illustration the social care practitioner is the leader supporting an African individual through dialogue and presence (see Table 5.1).

Table 5.1 Liberation techniques

Personal level	Leader level
Treat self with respect	Acknowledge that self-respect
Rest and relax	Affirm the importance of rest
Avoid negative rehearsals	Encourage pride on identity
Focus on positive performances	Praise and reinforce
Modelling identity pride	Express pleasure at progress made
Be pleased with self	Remain attentive, do not give up.

Source: adapted from Ruth 2006:141.

In addition to these techniques, he makes a helpful point in that leaders, in this case social care practitioners, need to get close enough to those that are feeling oppressed so as to be able to see and be touched by those things that are special about them, which they and others overlook or denigrate. It is important that social care workers get close enough to African families by allowing them to tell their stories, listen respectfully and empathize. From these stories, select expressions that can be used to affirm and encourage them to take pride in themselves as Africans living in the UK. Another aspect that makes some Africans feel bad about themselves, particularly women, is hair care as illustrated by this quotation:

> Nearly all my life, my mother has worn wigs. Though her own hair is short and somewhat thin, she has never experienced problems with balding or hair loss. She maintains that she is not very creative with her hairstyling and that wigs allowed her more styling options. What interests me is that even now as I reflect on these early years at home, the 1960s and 1970s is that neither my mother nor any of her many wig-wearing women friends owned afro or braided wigs, or wigs any-where close to black hairstyles and textures. Their wigs were always straight, long and flowing.
>
> (Lester 2000:202)

There is a great deal of wig-wearing and chemical treatment of hair to make it straight among African women. As mothers who are role models to their young daughters they may be unwittingly transmitting values about hair and beauty that would make their daughters dislike their natural curly hair leading to low self-esteem. For African children in care, the issue of hair and self-esteem is still around and does need to be addressed through dialogue and liberating techniques.

Summary

This chapter has provided insights into:

*   some of the pressures experienced by African families,
*   the process of change and transition individuals go through,
*   how internalized oppression can be counteracted towards liberation.

Exercise

1   Identify an African country that you know the least and research for information on family life in that country.
2   To search for information start with the British Council via their website: www.britishcouncil.org.

3 Search for information via the website of the country you have selected.

4 Compare the two sets of results and share your findings with your peers then discuss how you might use the evidence to support your engagement with African families going through transition and feeling racially oppressed.

6   Marriage patterns

This chapter will:

- discuss African marriage patterns,
- explore power dynamics within marriage,
- discuss possible implications in social care practice.

Marriage in Africa south of the Sahara

There are robust patterns in African marriage systems. Marriage in most African countries is a complex institution. The process may take several years, and follows a series of stages most of which are characterized by the performance of prescribed rites. For those who partake, these rites include integration of traditional African and Western family modes (Meekers 1992). Marriage is the joining together of two families, cementing a relationship between established groups. The marriage could be a monogamous or a polygamous union and both are common practice.

Another common practice that has remained constant over the years as part of a series of prescribed rites is the payment of agreed bride-wealth by one family to another: usually the husband's family makes the payment to the wife's family. Intense negotiations take place between representatives from each family. From these negotiations emerges an agreed bride-price with a time frame for payment.

This practice emerged as a significant feature among survey participants on social care with African families. While acknowledging that increased exposure to external influences may be diluting the practice, they confirmed that bride-price, bride-wealth or dowry, and transactions still occupy a position of cultural importance across most regions of Africa south of the Sahara.

Three statements cited below give a flavour of current thinking about this practice among the sample group members:

> Bride-price, sometimes referred to bride-wealth, is a payment of goods, money or livestock from the future son-in-law to the bride's parents.

Marriage payment is a way of establishing the coming together of two sets of families. The payment is also a way of securing the husband's rights over the children of that union.

(Practising social worker: participant (33))

What I do know is that bride-prices or dowries are given during a marriage, to secure recognition of marriage between the two persons. When this does not happen, it means the two people living together are not recognised as a married couple. This reflects on where their children belong and also on death, formal recognition of marriage determines inheritance protocol. Overall, marriage plays a significant role among Africans where ever they live.

(Student social worker: participant (4))

Bride-price is accepted as a natural thing that is expected, but, personally I hate the practice of bride price. Apart from making you feel like you are property of your in-laws, it also brings conflict within the home. From my experience, my ex-husband did not pay bride-price and because of that, I feel like my parents despise me even though I am the first born. My younger sister is respected because her husband paid a huge bride-price. Every time, they seek only her advice on most family issues and that hurts.

(Student social worker: participant (13))

From these statements, it would appear that the payment of bride-wealth remains a common practice as part of marriage systems among Africans who are living at home in Africa and/or abroad suggesting that those entering into marriage are likely to find it difficult not to conform to such a common practice even if their place of residence is the UK. What is also interesting is that Christianity does not allow the payment of bride-price and that most Africans living in the UK are practising Christians and yet they still see the need to engage in bride-price arrangements. These tensions have been around from the time when missionaries first went to Africa with a view to convert the Africans to Christianity. There have been differing views as to the benefits of bride-price payment ever since, as illustrated by correspondence between Methodist church leaders in Southern Rhodesia in 1933, one African, one European. In communicating to his European colleague, the Africa leader wrote:

many of your correspondents understand very little, if anything at all of this great Bantu custom. Lobola (bride-wealth) as an institution was never meant for gain. It was a concrete way of binding two families together. [In seeking to limit it] those who are directing Native Affairs in this country may find that they have made a law which cannot be kept. So far as native marriages are concerned I find lobola to be right.

> I am not favouring lobola amongst Christian people. What I dislike is
> the idea of making Christianity by law. It is a Christian ideal that a
> woman is on the same level with the man. Why try to make natives
> adopt Christian ideals before they become Christians.
>
> (Ranger 1995:44)

This correspondence needs to be read and understood within the
context of the church missionary involvement in colonial Africa. The
Africa marriage so referred has endured and continues to present day. Back
then, in the 1930s, the letter states bride-wealth was never meant for gain.
This remains a disputed position among opposing commentators. When-
ever transactions take place there are gains to be had on either side. Who
gains and by how much is determined by agreed protocol. African marriage transactions are meant to be of benefit to two sets of families, with
male members within those families benefiting the most materially and
prestige. A summary of expressed views by survey participants about some
of the implications of the practice of paying bride-wealth in relation to
women and men involved in the union of marriage tells a story that has
significance in terms of how women and men may perceive their role and
status within an African marriage.

Summary of expressed views

From the views expressed in Table 6.1, it would appear that the man is in
a favourable position within the marriage and that the woman takes a subservient position within the union and therefore these arrangements are
likely to affect power dynamics within some African families. Power differ-
entials, while recognized, have not altered this African custom.

Obbo (1980:36), in her study of African women and their struggle for
economic independence, found that among the Luo people, the custom of
giving bride-wealth was the cornerstone of marriage, which, if tampered
with, would weaken the whole institution. Nangoli (1986) holds the same
view and thinks that this practice should be continued because it is a way
of showing respect and a thank you. This 'thank you' is directed towards
the father of the bride who gives away his daughter so that she becomes

Table 6.1 Expressed views on bride-wealth payment

Woman	Man
Lower status	Greater power over family decisions
Seen as a commodity	Authority and absolute power over wife
Must honour and respect husband	Head of household
Subordinate	Dominate
Cannot leave her husband	Can leave his wife

fully incorporated into her husband's lineage. There are variations in practices between countries and within countries. For example, in some communities marrying out of the social group is the expected norm. Members may not marry anyone who is a member of their own lineage, however remote the genealogical connection may be (Kevane 2004, Gelfand 1979, Beattie 1966).

It can be argued that in general terms, the custom of giving bride-wealth is essential for a valid customary marriage even though few customary marriages are formally registered within a given state. The transaction is also accepted by many Africans as symbolic, in that the communities involved get to know that the bride's family have publicly pledged a commitment to hand over their daughter to the groom's family.

Monogamy

Monogamous marriage that involves one man and one woman is based on statutory law, whereas a polygamous marriage that involves two or more wives is based on customary law. When the marriage ceremonies are complete, the place of residence for the couple is dependent on the type of society they inhabit. In patrilineal society, where the children take the father's line, the bride leaves her natal group to join her husband's group. Because of the loss of the economic contribution of the daughter as she joins her new family, the bride-wealth is expected to be substantial. This could involve money, livestock and other goods. However, in matrilineal society, the bride retains ties with the family into which she was born. The bride-wealth is smaller than that expected in patrilineal society. In Africa, marriages are cultural events and ceremonies are elaborate. Generally, there is no such thing as an invited guest list. The extended family members from both sides do attend to celebrate the union. The giving of substantial bride-wealth, the formalization of the contract of marriage through customary or statutory law, all are confirmed openly by an elaborate ceremony, and from then on the husband acquires the rights over the children of the union.

Kevane (2004:92) states:

> the importance of rights is particularly salient in most African societies, for the simple reason that one of the parties to the marriage, the young girl, typically has few rights over her own actions. For the young woman, marriage is about creation and transfer of her rights, and less about her voluntary entry into a contract to create a household.

This suggests an inferior and less powerful position, for which many women accept and support its continuation by preparing their daughters for a similar type of marriage until such a time when many more women select to challenge marriage based inferior status. The giving of bride-wealth, the issue of rights, obligations and associated responsibilities are given different interpretations within and outside Africa. Those in favour of the bride-wealth practice, see it as the appropriate thing to do in order for the woman and man to feel that they are truly married. The practice is not viewed as buying a wife. However, what is interesting to note is that the transaction happens between men, and men are the beneficiaries of money, livestock and goods. It is not in their interest for those who benefit from the transaction to change it.

However, in history there have been women who objected to the giving of bride-wealth and broke with tradition because they considered the practice to be oppressive and made women depend on men for recognition, status and prestige. Among such women includes Buchi Emecheta, a well known woman who broke with tradition.

She was born 1944 in Lagos, Nigeria. It is reported that as a young woman of marriageable age, Buchi decided to go against the grain and refused the suitors that the family proposed and married a man of her choice. She also refused the traditional bride-price, because she believed that she should be able to meet her needs (Schwarz-Bart 2003). In this case it seems that her self-belief enabled her to challenge custom and tradition, migrate to the UK, where she faced many more challenges that she dealt with head on, to become an established author. This illustrative example provides evidence of how individuals have the capacity to fight internalized oppression by freeing themselves from the invisible cage in order to self-liberate. For now the jury is still out. Like Buchi Emecheta, some African feminists have challenged the practice of giving bride-wealth, because they consider the practice to be oppressive to women and affords power to men over women. According to the Women and Law in Southern Africa Research Trust (WLSA) (2001:207), the marriage payments legalize marriage, and as such the legal personhood of a woman upon marriage is usually compromised as she changes her identity and assumes that of her husband and in the process loses some of her rights.

In Southern Africa, men initiate the marriage process, have the power to make important decisions, rendering women powerless as encapsulated within the following narrative.

> A woman's sole right is to have no rights. She has no real power, only a pseudo-power. She can act, insofar as she causes no embarrassment to her husband. She can exist, insofar as she does not upset the capitalist system, thus, any power she may think she possesses is an illusion.
>
> (Thiam 1986:15)

While these views were expressed in a study conducted over twenty-five years ago, Africa remains a man's continent. Men across Africa south of the Sahara, hold all influential positions, politically, economically, some practice polygamy, remain heads of households within marriage, continue to pay bride-wealth and make decisions on succession and inheritance (SARDC-WIDSAA 2000, Kevane 2004). Perhaps any power women think they have is still an illusion. To illustrate further, the gender specific power positions between African women and men, IRIN humanitarian news analysis 17 July 2007 reported that daughters had become a high priced commodity in Zimbabwe. The report provided an example of a man who betrothed his fifteen year old daughter to a polygamous man thirty years her senior. The young woman became a fourth wife, but the arrangement did not last long because she ran away and sought refuge. In Zimbabwe children under the age of eighteen are minors, therefore, theoretically they are protected in law. This example shows that custom and tradition have yet to catch up with the national legal requirements in relation to the legal age for marriage in Zimbabwe. In this case, the head of household exercised his power and married off his daughter.

What power did the young woman's mother exercise to stop the unlawful marriage proceedings? Her low status position in her own marriage might provide the answer. However, it is likely that this young woman would behave differently and not accept a powerless position, given that she had the courage to escape to a place of safety. Change is possible if the oppressed group speak out and challenge the status quo. Because some women and men still take different positions on the issue of bride-wealth it can be argued that it is up to women to take a stand and involve men who wish to see social change. Among survey participants, social work students expressed different views on the issue of bride-price. For illustration, two contrasting views are noted below. The first one is by a male participant and the second by a female participant.

> I was raised by a father who had utmost respect to his wife. He told me that bride-price was not a form of purchasing a woman but a token of respect for the in-laws. Bride-price was meant to strengthen relationships between two families.
>
> (Social work student: participant (15))

> When the man is able to pay high bride-price, it gives him the absolute power to dominate the woman. Sometimes, the man will stay at home while the woman struggles to make ends meet for the family and in a sense, the woman becomes a slave.
>
> (Social work student: participant (31))

These two Africans, both young, would need to find a way to reconcile their differences and find common ground towards effecting change, if that is what is required. The evidence from existing literature and survey responses suggest that the practice of giving bride-wealth is still a common practice among most Africans, and that differences exist in interpretation of purpose and values behind the practice. But as with many traditions and customs in society, they do not remain static, change is inevitable. There are signs that the custom of giving bride-wealth is changing, be it slowly. Level of formal education, economic activity, equality legislation and women's campaigns for equal rights with men are influencing the formation of new cultures or making adaptations to the existing ones (Mvududu and McFadden 2001).

Some of those who take the view that bride-wealth benefits men and oppresses women, have referred to issues such as reproduction and inheritance.

> The issue of bride-wealth is often cited by men as an argument to control women's reproductive capacity. Men claim that since they pay bride-wealth, their wives belong to them and hence the control in marriages, despite the fact that marriage is a partnership. Male control within a marriage does not end with the wives; in most countries in the region men also have control over minor children in and/or out of marriage.
>
> (Southern African Research and Documentation Centre (SARDC) 2000:51)

Similarly, power to make decisions on inheritance after the death of a husband is biased in favour of men. In most countries with customary law women have no power over marital property, therefore women and their daughters do not inherit the deceased's property (Kevane 2004, Owen 1996, Obbo 1980). Those who wish to see change in the practice of giving bride-wealth argue that the practice commodifies women, affords them lower status and exclude them from important decisions relating to African family life, and as such keep more women in poverty than men and yet 70 per cent of food production is done by women (Amadiume 2000).

Polygamy (multiple wives)

According to Nangoli (1986), polygamy in Africa is accepted as a stabilizing instrument within the family. He suggests that African men as decision makers are of the firm belief that men, unlike their women folk, are naturally incapable of sustaining one relationship at a time. For this reason, it is thought that having multiple wives is better than having multiple extra marital relationships. However, the extent to which women accept the polygamous nature of men is open to debate and interpretation.

> African women seem to accept the polygamous nature of men and would not necessarily expect to live constantly with their husbands as most European wives do or demand standards of fidelity which they

would feel to be hypocritical. In this situation a woman may feel much freer to pursue her own interests and for instance to go abroad and study for several years, leaving the children in the care of co-wives or her own mother.

(Ellis 1978:24)

It seems as if the acceptance is in part influenced by the likely perceived benefits that can be accrued by being part of a polygamous marriage because women are free to fend for themselves and their children without having to wait in expectation that the husband will provide for all the co-wives and their children.

Available literature suggests that multiple wives remain a feature in Africa, and that there are variations in rates and views across the continent. The variations in rates are dependent on situational factors such as the level of industrialization, Western style development and women's level of formal education, in particular higher education. Some women accept this type of marriage as a normal customary practice, others think that it is a marriage system that is out of step with the social and economic demands of the modern world (Stacey and Meadow 2009). Hayase and Liaw (1997) view polygamy not only as a type of marriage, but a value system that has been resistant to the competition of an imported ideology of monogamy. Linked to a polygamous marriage system is the issue of reproduction where by traditionally it is argued that men needed multiple wives and children to work the land. Urbanization, education and paid employment opportunities have reduced the need for maintaining high levels of fertility, thus taking care of the economic argument. Missionaries and Christianity achieved some successes in promoting monogamy. These influences have been accompanied by a decline in polygamous unions. However, the value system has taken a new form such as 'outside wives' (Kevane 2004, Borgerhoff *et al.* 2001, Mann 1984, Ellis 1978).

By world standards, the incidence of polygamy in Africa south of the Sahara is considered to be high and commentators offer various reasons for the continuation of this form of marriage.

In their study on the state of polygamy in Africa (Hayase and Liaw 1997) estimated the percentages shown in Table 6.2. They justified their use of estimates because obtaining accurate figures is difficult if not impossible because very few customary marriages are registered. Another estimation is that the incidence of polygamous unions is lower among well educated women and men, but, among some well educated men, it is

Table 6.2 The state of polygamy

West Africa	40–50%
East Africa	20–30%
Southern Africa	10–15%

common for them to have socially recognized mistresses (Kevane 2004). Overall, the estimated percentages suggest that polygamous unions are part of the African cultural landscape and as such it is likely to be around for some years to come.

The practice of polygamy continues in African societies, possibly because some women and men do want to be involved in such unions because that is all they know; some women and men choose this type of union because they can do so legally; others do so out of necessity. However, the demands for gender equality in Africa will undoubtedly influence the nature and pace of change towards monogamous systems of marriage. Formal education is likely to have the biggest impact on polygamy in Africa south of the Sahara. Hayase and Liaw (1997) found that in Kenya and Zimbabwe women with higher education, the proportion of polygamy is reduced to zero. Economic independence that comes with higher qualifications improves their bargaining power about the choice of marriage system. Among African people living in the UK, and having connection with Africa, it means that they would have had first hand experience of the different marriage systems as daughters, sons, parents or grandparents. On migration, they are likely to have brought with them internalized social values and ideals relating to their kinship institutions. As such, bride-wealth practice is continued among some Africans who get married in this country. For some, the husband is the head of household and the wife plays a supportive role. Within some African households equality within marriage remains aspirational. The conflicts that arise as a result of exposure to the new culture and efforts to maintain and uphold African traditions could be contributing to a rising divorce rate among African couples living in the UK. The disproportionate number of African children in the care system could be partly attributed to the power dynamic difficulties in some African households. Difficulties and family problems can lead to the individuals concerned to connect with social care services for support. Therefore, those social care practitioners who are likely to be working with such families in difficulty can make use of some of this background information to assist with formulating useful questions that can facilitate meaningful engagement with users of the service.

Domestic violence against women is a taboo subject in Africa. Women are expected to put up with it and not to talk about the abuse outside the home. In the SARDC region, statistics on domestic violence show an increase, but commentators indicate that the figures are only a tip of the iceberg. It is suggested that women do not report violations for fear of ridicule and being castigated by family (SARDC 2000). It is unlikely that living in the UK makes all African women safe from domestic violence.

> Husbands beat their wives to either discipline them, or because they lose their temper. In both cases, the core of the problem is that women and men have different and changing expectations towards marriage,

family and intimate relationships and that, men are asserting and women are resisting masculine power to control women.

(SARDC 2000:163)

The available evidence suggests that African families living here draw on their customs and traditions to enable them to negotiate their path within the new culture. Retention and maintenance of some traditions such as giving bride-wealth can complicate equal partnership arrangements within marriage. The dominant position of most African men within households that is prevalent in Africa and has been internalized by those who have migrated to the UK, can lead some men to abuse their power and become violent towards their wives. Because there is a tradition in Africa of keeping domestic violence behind closed doors, some women do not take advantage of the UK systems of support. This is an area that requires attention and social workers play a part by working alongside African women's groups.

Summary

This chapter has provided insights into:

- African marriage processes,
- the extent and impact of polygamous unions,
- explored possible implications for the payment of bride-wealth.

Exercise

1 What is bride-wealth?
2 List your views about this system of marriage.
3 Identify the values implicit in your listed views.
4 How might these values influence your working relationship with African families?

7 Family and child rearing practices

This chapter will:

- discuss African family patterns,
- explore roles and responsibilities within family units,
- describe child rearing practices.

There are varied interpretations of what constitutes a family. The family can be thought of as a social institution set up to perform various functions (Leslie 1982). Leslie goes on to elaborate that a social institution is a system of social norms with regard to rules of conduct for its members. The rules of conduct are introduced to new members through the process of socialization, thereby learning the culture of a given society. These ideas would apply to the various countries that make up modern day Africa. There is likely to be a diversity of rules of conduct across the continent to reflect size of the geographical land mass. Scott (2001:48) offers his view indicating that institutions are social structures that have attained a high degree of resilience. The family would meet the resilience criteria despite modifications and the changes that have occurred within the last century. However, Giddens (2006) suggests that in some remote regions in Africa, traditional family systems are little altered. I would argue that these remote regions are likely now to be a minority because changes have been occurring since the beginning of the twenty-first century and many more African people have access to international information via cell phone network systems. Some of the changes relating to family systems in Africa are linked to new attitude formation as highlighted by Mvududu and McFadden (2001:74) in their WLSA study on reconceptualizing the African family in Southern Africa. WLSA studies show that there can be no one definition of the family – families exist which reflect the diverse and ever changing relationships through which identity, rights, entitlements, resources and power are contested, negotiated and distributed or accessed.

Among the many functions performed by the family within the framework of the ever changing relationships, they could be classified into four units, namely: reproduction, socialization of children, economic cooperation and common residence. How such functional units are organized is dependent on cultural norms. Functionalists, according to Giddens (2006), have regarded the nuclear family as fulfilling certain specialized roles in modern societies. Such a nuclear family would be composed of two adults living together in a household with their children. The nuclear family has become the norm in Western countries because the demands of modern industrialized societies are best served by such an arrangement of family life. Advocates of the nuclear family see it as the ideal in family living.

> Even in its weakened contemporary condition, the intact two-parent family committed to survival as a functional institution still performs better than any other variation as an agent for rearing responsible, healthy, adequately educated children, and a means of protecting the life, health, and happiness of adults.
>
> (Carlson 1993:46)

However, this idealized family remains just that, because such families only comprise less than 70 per cent of UK households. What is true is that the extended family is not the norm either. An extended family being a group of persons directly related by keen connections and this group may include grandparents, sisters and their husbands, brothers and their wives, aunts and uncles (Giddens 2006). In Africa extended families are the norm. Historically, African extended families could be subdivided in two ways: from one perspective, there was the division between the nucleus formed by the consanguineal core group and their children and the 'outer group' formed by the in-marrying spouses. African extended families may also be divided into their constituent conjugally based family units made up of parents and children McAdoo (1988). The extended nature of African family as it might be viewed by many Africans is best summed up by the following quotation:

> The family is not easy to define: in one sense the word can be used to include all persons living or dead, with a common ancestor, but generally the term extended refers to a group of closely related people known by a common name and consisting usually of a man and his wives and children, his sons' wives and children, his brothers and half-brothers and their wives and children, and probably other near relatives, all of whom are bound to each other by ties of mutual obligation.
>
> (Ellis 1978:16)

The inclusion of wives and half-brothers in this interpretation indicates an acceptance of polygamous marriages as discussed in the previous chapter. This definition implies a complex network of relationships, and individuals unfamiliar with such elaborate connections have to use their imagination in order to gain clarity about who is connected to who and the meaning of each link. Three aspects worthy of note about the African family are (Logan 1996):

- blood ties are very important,
- extended takes precedence over nuclear family,
- polygamous families are still quite common.

As with any institution there are advantages and disadvantages to this type of family in twenty-first century Africa and among African families who migrate to the UK and remain connected to this complex network of relationships. Among some of the advantages that have been documented the emphasis is skewed towards communal living to include day care for working mothers and social security and other welfare provisions that are essential for living because African countries do not have welfare states. According to Harden (1990), some African academics take a view that there is no alternative to the extended family in Africa, and that its functioning is a major way to distinguish African society from that of Europe or the United States. However, there are notable disadvantages to the African extended family which have become much more significant as Africa industrializes and people adopt monetary based lifestyles. It means that those with financial resources are expected to send remittances to members of their extended family to meet the costs of their living. When remittances fail to meet expectations this can lead to squabbles and a breakdown in harmonious relationships. The stresses brought on by unrealistic expectations from a large number of relatives is making some people, particularly the emerging middle class, question the wisdom of continuing with traditional family systems, while attempting to industrialize using Western style techniques and methods. Perhaps an African nuclear family is the way forward if Western styles of living become the norm. This arrangement of family life would enable those Africans living abroad to focus attention on their immediate family, thereby reducing feelings of guilt for not sending remittances 'back home' to Africa.

Another change worthy of note within African families is the fact that interracial unions are on the increase, particularly among Africans living abroad and/or their offspring. Some Africans who migrated to the UK or their offspring married interracially. This trend is likely to continue suggesting that social care publications about African families living in the UK need to include issues that are thought to be important and may have implications for policy and practice. One of the issues that has been debated within social care circles over the past two decades relates to mixed race children received into the local authority care system. Some of these children may have African/European parents. Based on the Department of Health Adoption Register (2003), there is evidence to suggest an overrepresentation of mixed race children in the care system and that these children are underrepresented in adoption placements (Frazer and Selwyn

2005). Poverty and relationship breakdown are some of the reasons for their reception into the care of local authorities. Their reception into care makes it necessary that all those people involved in their care are meaningfully engaged with issues affecting mixed race children, and identity is one of those issues that should not be ignored in view of the earlier discussion on African traditional customs and family systems.

In her research findings, Ifekwunigwe (1999:17) reflected on the fact that mixed race people themselves, as well as parents, carers, practitioners, educators, policy makers, academics and curious laypeople, are all hungry for a uniform but not essentialist term that creates a space for the naming of their specific experiences without necessarily re-inscribing and reifying race. Informal and formal conversations with myriad mixed race people have also demonstrated that to date we have not found a way to formulate discourses that do not re-inscribe a dominant binary black/white mixed race paradigm.

Ten years have passed since her publication and the hunger is yet to be satisfied.

Barn and Harmon (2006) confirms that the development of racial and ethnic identity of minority ethnic children and young people in the UK remains an important academic area of concern. The development of racial and ethnic identity has implications for mixed African/European families. The academic and professional concern on the subject matter would suggest the need for appropriately funded ongoing research because the composition and structure of the UK population will continue to change and, with those changes, it is likely that societal attitudes will also change.

As highlighted in Chapter 1, Africans have been coming to the UK for the past two centuries. Some settled and married local Europeans and raised their children successfully by local standards. There have been others, who fathered children but did not commit to marriage and returned to their countries of origin leaving the children behind with their mothers. Research shows that a high number of children in care come from a family headed by a lone white mother and of this high number, a significant proportion will have absent black fathers, some of whom are African (Barn 1999). Some of these children were taken into local authority care for a variety of reasons. However, among African/European families who remain in the UK and make a success of their relationships there are often no issues of concern, therefore social workers do not get involved. These families establish their own ways of parenting their mixed race children. Perhaps lessons could be learnt from those who make a success of mixed race relationships and more importantly their parenting styles, given that the social construction of race is embedded in the psyche of the majority of the UK population. More often than not, polarized debates focusing on identity have tended to focus on failures.

A recent investigation for the Joseph Rowntree Foundation into parenting mixed race children elicited the views of parents and children on issues of belonging, identity and cultural differences (Caballero *et al.* 2008). It was established that for the sample group, parents adopted different approaches that were categorized into three approaches to parenting, namely, an individual, a mix and a single approach. In summary the key elements for each approach are:

- in a single approach, one aspect such as religion informs family rules and values,
- in a mixed approach, acknowledgement of specific heritages and mixedness regarded as an identity in and of itself,
- in an individual approach, cosmopolitan lives are acknowledged and children enabled to feel free to make choices about their identities.

The conclusion was that there is no one best way that parents can understand their children's identity. If local authorities in their corporate parenting role were to give some attention to the ideas emerging from this research, they would need to figure out an approach they would adopt for its family of mixed race children given that mixed race children are over-represented in the care system and are underrepresented in adoption placements. Because this was a small scale study, critics will undoubtedly raise questions about representativeness and reliability. What is needed is a well funded representative study on parenting mixed race children. The results could move the debate forward as well as establishing where families and their children are at in present day UK.

Some of the existing literature on ideological positions has influenced social work policy and practice in relation to mixed race children. The issue of language and labelling has been debated by social care practitioners and policy makers, going as far back as the previous Conservative government of the 1980s. During this period, same-race placements of children became the preferred option. The variety of labels that were used to describe children born to parents from different races included for example: mixed race, dual heritage or multiple heritage.

This labelling can be viewed as emphasizing a sense of being different from the rest of the children whose parents belong to the same race category. Problems can arise if the differences are highlighted negatively in an exclusionary way or when young people of interracial parentage are treated as a homogeneous group. However, if the label is used to support service planning and delivery of relevant and appropriate care for each young person, this can be positive. The best judges of positivity would be the users of the service. Ideological positions have informed the development of two competing perspectives: the black perspective and the mixed perspective. Both have a part to play because they reflect the complexity of the politics of race and the real and ever changing world in which social care practitioners must exercise professional judgements affecting other people's lives.

The black perspective can be linked back to the 1970s and 1980s anti-racist discourse (Barn and Harman 2006, Tizard and Phoenix 1993). Influenced by the debates stimulated by the association of black social workers and allied professions on transracial placements of children during the 1980s the issue of black identity came to the fore. The arguments in favour of an emphasis on a black identity for mixed race children in local authority social services care were that society viewed mixed race children as black. By reinforcing the child's black heritage, this would support those providing care to find ways of ensuring that young people in the care of a local authority have the knowledge and skills to deal with the effects of racism. The black perspective gives attention to how it is believed that a mixed race young person will be seen by society at large. But some critics of the black perspective see it as rigid and inflexible thereby contradicting the notion that people should be free to define their own identity and ignores the research that shows mixed race young people with a positive identity, and also failure to acknowledge potential for prejudice and bigotry from within the black community has been raised as an issue of concern (Barn and Harman 2006). Among some black people who subscribe to this perspective, they see themselves as having the interests of the child at the centre the debate, and very often their ideas will have been shaped by their observed or first hand experience of racism and discrimination. For some Africans, the history of domination and colonization would influence their thought processes and the stance they would take on issue of identity when it comes to child rearing.

The mixed perspective highlights the importance of self-determination because self-labelling empowers those who select their own labels. It opposes black identity as the only correct identity for mixed race children. Multiple heritages are acknowledged, the one drop of blood rule is rejected, therefore identification with both parents is considered to be important. For example children with African/European parents would identify with both sides of their racial heritage.

Critics of the mixed perspective (Maxime 1993, Small 1993), suggest that politicized black identity opposition confirms the theory that blackness is negative hence the need to neutralize its impact. Similar to the rigidity associated with a black perspective; there is also a danger of denying self-definition among those mixed race young people who see themselves as black due to their particular set of circumstances and lived experience.

These two competing perspectives around issues of identity have points of convergence in that the welfare of children remains central to the debate and that the construction of race continues to have a negative impact on young people in the UK. This convergence can influence ongoing critical reflection among practitioners and social policy makers in order that they can identify how and what to assess and subsequently inform the nature of selected intervention. Both perspectives have a part to play and need to be accommodated if young people from interracial families are to be appropriately supported. How each young person received into the local authority social care system sees itself should be the starting point in planning care. Graham (2007) emphasizes the importance of listening to children and giving attention to children's narratives of their lived experience. The legal framework provides a basis from which both perspectives can be incorporated when arranging an individualized care package. The 1989 Children Act, Section 22, makes specific reference to children from minority communities, acknowledging their presence and placing a legal requirement to consider a child's racial, cultural, religious and linguistic background in the care and provision of services. The minority status of people of interracial parentage was officially confirmed through the 2001 census with population figure of 661,034. This is a significant minority population, from which some young people may end up in the care system and for whom appropriate placements would need to be found to enable these young to realize their potential. Self-definition/classification seems to be the favoured position. Internationally recognized political figures in significant positions of authority such as the president of the United States of America whose mixed race parentage is well publicized is reported by some media outlets to be the first African/American president and some media refer to Mr Obama as the first black president, perhaps the one drop rule applies as highlighted by proponents of the black identity perspective. I guess self-identification does apply to the president of the USA.

Roles and responsibilities within African families

In most African households the mother has responsibility for childcare arrangements, all the domestic work and ensuring that the family is clothed and has enough to eat. She is the 'mum in chief' to use Mrs Obama's expression. A woman is accepted as the essence of being and existence because she bears children. Generally all adult women are regarded as mothers and peacemakers.

The father is the leader who overseas all family activities and makes all the major decisions about family life. He is responsible for creating a homestead for his wife or wives, but variations exist between countries, communities and groups. Children have responsibility for undertaking age specific tasks set for them, and must do so willingly as a way of showing respect to their parents. When they become adults they have a responsibility towards their parents and provide social security. From the outset, children are seen as an insurance policy for their parents. Grandparents have a responsibility for officiating at family ceremonies and for sorting out disputes. They use their knowledge and wisdom to advise the younger generation and, as such, they have an important educational role within a given community and are afforded corresponding respect (Kevane 2004, Nangoli 1986, Gelfand 1979).

Child rearing practices

Survey results on issues relating to child rearing practices familiar to African student social workers seemed to suggest that their responses were based on first hand experience because of the way in which the narratives were presented. There were expressions of what it had been like for them when they were growing up as well as sharing some of their thoughts that stemmed from the exposure in their communities. Because of that recent lived experience, their views could inform social care thought in planning for, and when interacting with, African families. The following selected examples represent the views of the majority.

> Children are every adult's responsibility. Respect for all adults is also considered to be mandatory. However, with so much talk about freedom of expression with regard to relationships, parents can be quite wary about enforcing respect indiscriminately; choosing instead to safeguard the children against liberal culture.
>
> (Student social worker: participant (1))

> Although the child has got its biological father and mother to provide and support it financially and to meet the child's basic needs, others chip in. The child according to most African cultures does not belong exclusively to the biological parents, but belongs to the whole community. Everyone in the community have a duty to raise the child. They help in shaping the child's character.
>
> (Student social worker: participant (24))

> Fostering practice – child rearing that allows upbringing to be shared among the extended family members. This child-rearing practice urges all to protect the child's health and welfare and ensures its safety. It is a practice I have grown up with.
>
> (Practising social worker: participant (19))

> In Africa a child could live with parents and in the absence of parents, a child could live with a relative who would help bring up the child as if it were their own. Sometimes a child could live with non relatives who would receive payment.
>
> (Student social worker: participant (7))

The pattern that emerges is one of shared responsibilities for childcare within a given community, including kinship foster care. Perhaps this goes back to economics and social insurance, in that well looked after children are likely to thrive to become adults who will take on the responsibility of looking after elderly parents. Other practices that seemed distinctive to Africans is the length of a breast feeding period, thought to be twelve

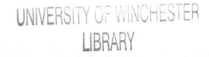
UNIVERSITY OF WINCHESTER
LIBRARY

months for most people. Bonding and attachment is promoted through the way in which infants and toddlers are transported, nearly always on the back of their mothers. The importance of obedience and respect was noted by all the participants suggesting that these practices are observed by Africans in the UK.

By drawing on what they know now and have experienced recently, the participants concurred with findings from earlier studies on African child rearing practices (Evans and Myers 1994, Fuller and Toon 1988, Ellis 1978, Gelfand 1979, Beattie 1966).

Africans living in the UK continue to subscribe to these practices as far as it is possible to do so. But in certain situations the practice may contravene UK legislative norms. For example, parents are accountable and responsible for the upbringing of their children and not the extended family members or the whole community. Informal kin foster care arrangements without social services suitability assessment would raise safeguarding issues. Older children would not be expected to look after younger siblings without the supervision of their parents. 'Latch key kids' arrangements are not acceptable.

Child discipline

Survey results show that Africans expect their children to be obedient, respectful and as such consequences of bad behaviour would always be explained. Involving other people associated with the family to talk to children about unacceptable behaviour seems to be an acceptable method that produces positive results for some. Perhaps the idea that in Africa it takes a village to raise a child, has been transported by some families who try to continue a similar practice in the UK.

Illustrative statements include: 'Africans appear to discipline their children by training them to know the limits of their behaviour – what is acceptable and what is not. This may mean being firm, in control, offer explanations, offer praise and reward as appropriate' (practising social worker: participant (29)).

> I smack my children. I do not let the government come in my house to discipline my children. I only do smack when it's really necessary, but mostly I talk to them and try to show them the outcomes of their actions.
> (Student social worker: participant (10))

> I don't think that Africans have a choice on this one other than to stick with the UK laws. I was raised understanding that if my mischief was grave enough to deserve a good beating I would certainly deserve one. Most Africans can no longer implement this kind of discipline for fear of losing them to social services.
> (Student social worker: participant (18))

This area has seen a marked transition and there is demonstrated awareness that physical chastisement is not acceptable. Children might still be shouted at but there will be a lot of negotiations, a stronger attempt to win over though mostly they will be grounded for a period of time. As an extreme measure, parents will threaten and even contemplate taking them back to Africa to stay with relatives.

(Practising social worker: participant (3))

Key themes to emerge around child discipline are categorized into sub-headings in Table 7.1.

The narratives around each of the themes appear to suggest that some African families work with change constantly adapting and adjusting their methods of discipline in response to the social and legal demands of the environment in which they live. The responses to this question were directly connected to how African families living in the UK are disciplining their children, rather than current practices in Africa. The highlighted practices are not that dissimilar to the common practices instituted by the majority of parents here. What is probably different and has been implemented by some African-Caribbean parents is the idea of short stays abroad in order to be exposed to other ways of living with the view that travel broadens the mind and hopefully on return to the UK the children will be better behaved and appreciative of parental availability. The African regions represented by the participants cover a significant geographical area, namely, West, Central, East and Southern Africa. For specific names of the countries represented refer to Chapter 1. The diversity of cultures is to be expected across the continent, but common threads often run through them. For example, the culture in terms of raising children is linked to what Africans consider being important and is valued as indicated by the results from the survey. One such thread is that African children are expected to show respect for their elders by the way they communicate, verbally or non-verbally. The issue of respect was identified to be significant as far back as the late 1970s but still holds true today. Ellis (1978:18) stated, however alien it may seem to our society with its emphasis both on youth and on individual freedom, that understanding the significance of respect for one's elders is one of the keys to the understanding of

Table 7.1 Child discipline categories and techniques

Communication	Isolation
Talk	Withdraw privileges
Explain	Restrict outings with friends
Involve others	Boundaries
Praise	Short stay in Africa
Telling off	Grounding

African societies. The young, well educated, well dressed woman who kneels to her elders, and the young graduate who prostrates to his illiterate mother, are showing respect without the subservience that such behaviour would convey to the British.

Thirty years on, have these forms of showing respect changed? The answer is yes in that modifications do happen over time and new ways of respecting elders are introduced. What has remained constant is the relevance and importance of showing respect to one's elders. Therefore, respect for adults within African communities cannot be overemphasized. Children are not expected to talk back to adults in African societies, but to respond in prescribed ways when spoken to. Overall the African centred values that emphasize a sense of connectedness, interdependency and collective responsibility underpins child rearing practices.

The extent to which African child rearing practices can be taken into account by professional practitioners responsible for the care of African children is a debate that needs to be had. A study of ethnic minority families, including African families, found that respect for elders and child discipline was similar among all minority families (Beishon *et al.* 1998). Ten years on, the African student social workers survey supports the findings of the earlier study, suggesting that positive common practices could be shared, for the benefit of all.

Management responsibility for change

There is evidence to suggest that there are black African children in the local authority care system, and that their parents have origins in Africa south of the Sahara. The specificities of African children's experiences in the care system are unknown. Normal African family life in the UK has rarely been studied.

(Kyambi 2005)

Such gaps in knowledge are likely to have an impact on decision making about safeguarding African children. For changes to happen managers need to support staff in knowledge acquisition about African children and their families, as stakeholders should be involved in sharing their lived experiences with all the agencies that have a responsibility for safeguarding children. The agencies are required under government legislation to work closely together. This is because the investigations into a number of child deaths showed that one of the major failures is that social services departments and other agencies failed to communicate and work together in ways that would protect children (Henderick 2003). The evidence has led to the creation of a safeguarding board in each local authority with the responsibility of ensuring that the agencies work together so as to ensure that all children in their localities are kept safe.

In addition to these structures, there is a greater push for service users to be consulted and to participate in decision making, thereby, providing a window of opportunity for African families receiving social care services to be consulted. However, it is recognized that there are difficulties around real participation of service user. These must be acknowledged in order that they can be addressed. Glasby (2007) argues that although there is a growing influence of people who use public services, there is still a concern that there is little meaningful involvement. As a result, the criticism is one of tokenism. If African users of social care services are to be involved, tokenism is to be avoided otherwise no meaningful progress could be achieved. Managers can take a strategic view and find answers to questions that are likely to arise about the nature and level of service user involvement while safeguarding children. For example, if African families need services that are not in line with organizational policy, how will this be managed?

If an African community group was contracted to run a social care service, would the service still be provided to the standard required by social services? Who would take responsibility when things go wrong? How much would the change in practice cost? Through raising such questions, clarifications can result (Aldgate *et al.* 2007). The results of the student survey indicated that African children do rarely speak up in the presence of adult relatives, so their involvement would need careful thought.

Local authorities have policies that have been formulated in response to the shift from welfare models of provision to one that promotes well-being and inclusion needs that are underpinned by effective engagement of those who use services to help shape the design, delivery and monitoring service quality. Because this way of working is increasingly being adopted and enabling users to be meaningfully involved, there is a window of opportunity to engage African families.

One way to involve African children, who have a care protection plan, would be the creation of a supportive group of young people so that the members can share their experiences away from adults. With the support of family social care workers, the children can express their concerns about the service and discuss possible solutions. African children need to be heard. It is part of a manager's job working in children services to ensure active service user involvement, by giving separate spaces to parents and children. Reasons for the separate approach would need to be made clear to parents. As highlighted earlier, African children are unlikely to speak up in front of their parents or most adults without the use of specific directive approaches. However, their involvement is important to ensure appropriateness of service they receive.

Summary

This chapter has provided insights into:

- the nature of family patterns,
- child rearing practices,
- significant roles within the family,
- parental discipline,
- involving families and children meaningfully.

Exercise

1 What are the values that underpin childcare in Africa?
2 Do these values conflict with childcare practices in the UK?
3 How would you manage the conflict?

8   Religion and spirituality

This chapter will:

• examine the role of religion and spirituality,
• analyse the impact of religion on family life.

Religion forms part of ancient African traditions, and as such African religious traditions are complex and diverse to reflect the size of the continent and its peoples. Kamara (2000:504) puts forward a view that to be African is to be religious, to be alive is to be religious and to be religious is to work towards the enhancement of the community to please the Supreme Creator. The religious traditions provide a means of meeting spiritual needs and as such spirituality is integral to the way in which many Africans understand the world and their place in it (Nangoli 1986, Kamalu 1990, Karenga 1993, Ver Beek 2002).

From the views put forward by these authors, it would appear that in African religious traditions, there is a visible physical entity and an invisible world inhabited by the supernatural. Therefore, among those who subscribe to this worldview, the physical and the spiritual are intertwined and as such provide meaning that informs people's actions.

As a frame of reference in distilling this complexity into a manageable format, Karenga (1993:213) provides four distinctive themes that are highlighted as follows.

Theme one focuses on the idea of God: among believers, the supremacy of God guides their conduct in all aspects of their life. This God is viewed as male; therefore, the term father is used in most African societies.

Theme two considers God to be immanent and transcendent: this Supreme Being is both near and far. This aspect is demonstrated through the engagement with divinities that are seen as intermediaries.

Theme three gives attention to ideas around Ancestor veneration: ancestors are venerated as models of ethical life, and that they are intercessors between the human being and the Creator.

Theme four addresses individual and collective identity: in this regard, religion stresses the necessary balance between one's collective identity and has responsibility as a member of society. A person is defined as an integral part of a specific community.

In addition to the four general themes, Karenga (1993) acknowledges and refers to the work by Mbiti (1970), who highlights the importance of acknowledging the moral ideal of harmonious integration of self with the community and that the highest moral ideal is to live in harmony. Linked to harmonious living is an important value of respecting the natural world. In this regard, nature is respected for its association with God as well as its relevance to people and humanity. These ideas expressed thus far about community, harmonious living, respect for the environment and belief in God, do not contradict the principles of social care. It is therefore possible for social care practitioners in the UK to work effectively with families whose outlook on family life is influenced by African religious traditions.

The diversity and complexity of religious beliefs in Africa has been compounded further by external influences and, as such, some Africans who migrated to the UK are likely to have brought with them an outlook on family life that has been influenced by African religious traditions, their understanding of Christianity and Islam as they were introduced to them, and subsequently adapted and Africanized. Some of the evidence suggests that Christianity and Islam have a significant following in Sub-Saharan Africa (Gyimah *et al.* 2006). Christianity has two strands. One strand is Coptic Christianity that came out of ancient African religion and flourished in Ethiopia, Sudan and Egypt. The second strand is European Christianity that was introduced by missionaries from the North and has tended to remain tainted with cultural colonialism (Kamalu 1990).

This form of European Christianity spread through West, Central, East and Southern Africa in different circumstances within the context of colonial and settler power. The negative association is not about Christian religion per se, but the use to which it was put in subjugating the colonized to a new culture. Apart from Christianity, Islam is considered to have come from outside Africa. Islam was not the religion of the colonial power nor of Western education, and it has different international connection and its own particular formulations of the relations of sacred and secular power (Ranger 1986:1). Islam came to Africa from Arabia after the death of Muhammed in AD 632. It is claimed that the impact of Islam has been more widely felt than that of European Christianity, possibly because it is less remote from the African traditional way of life. The timing for the spread of Islam is linked to migration for economic trade.

> The primary reason for the success of Islam in Black Africa, with one exception, consequently stems from the fact that it was propagated peacefully at first by solitary Arabo-Berber travellers to certain Black kings and notables, who then spread it about them to those under their jurisdiction.
>
> (Diop 1987:163)

This initial contact between the travellers and the notables suggests a peaceful conversion to Islam prior to the introduction of the slave trade. It is estimated that between the seventh and ninth centuries Islam had covered North Africa and began to move southwards beyond the Sahara desert (Kamalu 1990). Kamalu points out that progressively the pattern of peaceful conversion changed, and his research suggests that Islam was then used by Arab slave traders and soldiers to subjugate Africans economically, politically, as well as to mould the African cultural personality into a form that is passive rather than resistant to Arab cultural domination. However, he is keen to point out that his criticisms are not about Islam as a religion, but the use to which it was put. Therefore, in a similar way to Christianity, Islam is a religion used by Arab slave traders and as such it is tainted with cultural domination. Examples of cultural domination include the adoption of Christian or Muslim names and the giving up of African names in order to fit in and to be allowed to participate fully within the new culture. In an attempt to retain some aspects of their traditions, African Christians and Muslims practise their religion in a way that is different to the way Europeans and Arabs practise. An Africanization of these religions continues to take place by incorporating elements of traditional worship such as vocalization, use of drums and rhythmic spiritual dance. Kamalu (1990:19) suggests that Christianity and Islam have been assimilated into the African personality, as opposed to the African personality assimilating a foreign culture.

All these religions have shaped and influenced patterns and forms of African family life. Historical European colonization of Africa means that the majority of the religious population is Christian with an Africanized dimension of faiths. Christians follow the teachings of various denominations such as Catholicism, Anglican, Methodism, Salvation Army and Pentecostalism. Islam has a following in some West African and East African countries. Examples of the impact of these religions on African family life include the roles and status of men and women, initiation ceremonies, marriage practices and formal education. It can be argued that externally introduced religions were used to capture the nature of new social formations among people who were experiencing the impact of capitalist modes of economic activity as well as different forms of political activity.

Ranger's (1995) historical research on the Samkange family shows how Methodism embraced by this family influenced their views of formal education, politics, monogamy and the status of women in Zimbabwe (then Southern Rhodesia). Across colonial Africa south of the Sahara, Christianity through mission schools has had a lasting effect on the nature and pace of change towards the adoption of European lifestyles including post-independence education policies. In his research on mission schools in Africa, Kallaway (2009:218) concluded that mission churches had a very significant influence on the shaping of educational thinking in the colonial and imperial context at a time when the state influence in the sector was still quite weak, but not all influences were helpful and positive. For example, on polygamy as a value system in Africa, recent research seems to suggest that Christianity has had a negative effect.

With respect to religion, Christianity with its negative moral judgement on polygamy has a clear negative effect on the polygamy propensity in all four countries (Senegal Ghana, Kenya, Zimbabwe). Of particular interest is the relatively

> high polygamous tendencies of the followers of the Spiritual religion in Zimbabwe. To the extent that this religion represents an adaptation of Christianity to traditional African values, we find that the Africans have become assertive in dealing with imported culture.
>
> (Hayase and Liaw 1997:324)

Against this backdrop, it can be argued that Christianity is still thriving in Africa and influencing decisions to retain some traditions and reject Christian teachings, adapt some to accommodate African values and/or adopt most of Western capitalist/socialist Christian teachings. Assumptions arising from this line of argument, is that most African Christians who migrated to the UK would be at ease with these Christian teachings. Dr Sentamu, the Archbishop of York, and the former Archbishop of Cape Town, in their capacity as public figures, can be viewed as representative of some Africans who have embraced Christianity and the corresponding theological teachings that are informed by the principles of social justice. They have both worked tirelessly to mobilize church support for a more just and equal society than that which is in place. However, critics of the way in which the majority of Africans have embraced Western Christianity and Islam suggest that Africans perceive their religion as inferior to other religions. This perception makes the few who practise African traditional religion, do so in secrecy to avoid embarrassment (Kamara 2000). Unfortunately, inferiority and secrecy while living in a foreign country can have negative consequences on family life among a minority of Africans living in the UK.

Definition of religion and spirituality

Generally, it is acknowledged that religion and spirituality are complex constructs. However attempts have been made to provide varied interpretations of meaning as illustrated by the following statements: 'Religion involves belief in spirituality, a divinely-based moral code, and seeing the purpose of life as increasing harmony in the world by doing good and avoiding evil' (Loewenthal and Cinnirelli 2003:112); 'Religion can be viewed as a social institution Concerned with the way beliefs, practices rituals and communities are organised, while spirituality concerns the individual quest to understand and attribute meaning to life and the sacred' (Ridge *et al.* 2008:414).

Ver Beek (2002:63) defines spirituality as a relationship with the supernatural or spiritual realm which provides meaning and a basis for personal and communal reflection, decisions and actions. He goes on to suggest that religion is associated with an institutionalized set of beliefs and practices linked to spirituality that has a bearing on the relational aspect of people's beliefs which shape their daily life.

Healy (2005) considers the meaning of religion to be a systematic body of beliefs and practices associated with spiritual search. Those who search, seek personal fulfilment. These interpretations of religion and spirituality highlight their importance among those people who subscribe to that way of life. It seems therefore necessary that social care practitioners need to acknowledge these aspects of people's beliefs and daily influences on their family life at the point of contact and subsequent interactions. To be certain about each individual family's religious affiliation, asking appropriate questions that do not cause embarrassment would ensure non-evasive appropriate response.

In African traditional religion, the human being is at the centre of the universe. Thus in moral terms, the human being is the route of all value (Kamalu 1990:14). The words and phrases within the above interpretations of religion and spirituality from different perspectives associated with different religions include search, purpose, fulfilment, morality, belief, divinely, doing good, and all can readily be associated with caring and empowerment values that inform social care practice. Similar words and phrases were echoed by survey participants in responding to the question on the role of religion among Africans living in the UK while confirming that religion played a significant role in family life given that most Africans are religious. Additionally their responses on the importance of religion concurred with Obomanu (2003:167), in which he states: 'the role of religion in the black family and community life remains more prominent than the increasingly secular modern white culture'.

Why this prominence among African people whose forebears were introduced to Western style Judeo-Christian traditions only a century ago? The answer might be found within the processes and experiences of migration. Migrant peoples usually take with them their religious beliefs and practices as something to hold on to while they adapt to a new environment. The church community can also provide social care for older people, childcare and parenting groups. The history of oppression and discrimination could be a factor. According to Ridge *et al.* (2008) many African individuals turned to religion to help them cope with difficult and at times traumatic life circumstances including illness, poverty and uncertain immigration status. It seems therefore that when people follow religious practices and associate with other believers they can draw strength from association and use that strength to help them to deal with negative experiences resulting from structural/institutional forms of oppression. The importance of religion among Africans living in the UK is illustrated in

Table 8.1 The role of religion in African family life

Identity	Friendship	Guidance	Inner strength
Solidarity	Solace/comfort	Seek advice	Coping mechanism
Togetherness	Well-being	Lifestyle	Healing
Common belief	Fearless	Survival	Comfort
Similarity	Recognition	Protection	Self-esteem
Trust	Association	Counselling	Hope

Table 8.1, based on a summary of responses from a survey of African students and practising social workers.

In Table 8.1, the role of religion in African family life is categorized into the four themes – identity, friendship, guidance and inner strength. It is noticeable that the words and phrases listed under each category are generally about construction and not destruction, suggesting that religion has a positive value among those who partake, in line with the definitions of religion stated on above. This positive value can be beneficial to practitioners when they are planning for social care interventions with African families that are known to belong to specific religious groups. It therefore requires that practitioners become comfortable in their dealings with families who subscribe to religious faiths, even if the practitioners are not religious. The social care value of respect for the individual should enable them to engage without too much discomfort as they are frequently called upon to try walking a 'mile' in someone else's shoes. Illustrative examples of full statements from survey participants about the importance of religion among Africans include:

> Religion plays a massive role because it brings Africans together when they attend church services. The church is one place where some Africans gather together, and through religion, community spirit is formed. Most associations formed by Africans have done so through religion. It is also a way for them to feel that they belong somewhere, in a foreign land. It gives most families a sense of social belonging and to be identified with as part of a social group in the community.
>
> (Practising social worker: participant (27))

> Church members can be part of an extended family, because most people who came to the UK left their extended families behind. So by going to church, it is hoped that it might provide that missing link. Having a faith provides a balance in life. Without it in the UK, one could be lost and lose values and identity.
>
> (Student social worker: participant (2))

> Very important, I try to take my children to church to impart religion and spirituality in them. However, the older children who have grown

up don't value religion as much as we did when we were growing up. Religion gives me hope and some thing to trust in.

(Student social worker: participant (4))

Religion plays quite a significant role. Due to being apart from their families, this is a source of security and inspires dependency on God and fellow black believers. However, due to financial burdens/responsibilities, total devotion to church attendance and/or other spiritual matters can be compromised.

(Practising social worker: participant (30))

These statements represent the views of the majority of survey participants indicating the prominence of religion among most Africans living in the UK. It is therefore likely that religion influences the way they conduct their family affairs. These findings about the importance of religion among Africans concur with the findings of an earlier study (Ridge *et al.* 2008) on the role of spirituality and religion for people living with HIV in the UK. The majority of Africans who participated in that study were found to be deeply religious and believed that they could hand over control of uncontrollable situations to the higher power of God.

These Africans attributed considerable credit to prayer for their wellbeing and good fortune. Perhaps disorientation as a result of migration and a sense of powerlessness make people feel the need to hand over control of the uncontrollable situations to the higher power of God who could intervene on their behalf. Social care practitioners working with African families who believe in handing over control of the uncontrollable situations to God through prayer would need to seek appropriate methods for intervention through faith groups and religious leaders. Faith group members and Church leaders are likely to have an understanding of their congregation memberships and be well placed to share with practitioners specific methods of engagement that are likely to have an impact with a view to achieve desired outcomes. However, it is important that professional skills, social care knowledge and the law are relied upon to decipher practices that are likely to work and produce positive results while ensuring that safeguarding issue are not compromised. This approach would involve practitioners in getting to know the communities they serve by undertaking research, profiling and locating the various African community and faith groups, their church leaders then deciding how, where and when interactions would take place.

Where do Africans meet for services and worship? African Christians attend their local denominational church such as: Methodist, Catholic, Church of England and Church of Scotland. Some Africans attend Pentecostal churches that come under the umbrella of Protestantism. This is where black people make up a sizeable proportion of the congregation. Pentecostalism puts an emphasis on ecstatic experience in prayer, where participants can verbalize freely in praise of God. African Muslims attend their local mosques together with other people whose origins are in different parts of the world. Evidence from various studies suggests that the majority of the African population across the continent is religious and make a significant contribution to the three billion people who use sacred texts in guiding the way they live their lives (Kim and Draper 2008, Takyi 2003, Patel *et al.* 2002). The sacred texts and religions influential among Africans living in the UK are listed below.

Protestantism

The rejection of authoritarian church structure and attention to individual conscience and faith has enabled the creation of a large number of Protestant groups, differing on various points of faith practice and church organization. However, these Protestant groups have much in common, such as the emphasis on the individual's direct relationship with God. Protestant groups have ministers, pastors and church elders who officiate and play a pastoral role in their communities. Black churches in the UK are part of the protestant community that has developed a bible based specific form of worship (Fuller and Toon 1988).

In urban areas such as London, Birmingham and Manchester it is not uncommon for Africans to attend all night prayer sessions at weekends led by a pastor. These sessions are vocally expressive and individuals feel that they can talk directly to God.

Catholicism

The Pope is the head of the Catholic Church worldwide based at the Vatican in Rome. The Bible provides the basis for all teachings and practices. Sacraments are important to practising Catholics and these sacraments are linked to specific signposts through life stages such as:

- birth
- baptism
- marriage
- anointment of the sick
- death.

Participants are expected to attend church, confess their sins to a priest and seek absolution. Use of contraception, and abortion of a foetus, remain controversial within families and the church community, and can lead to internal and intra-familial conflicts.

Church of England/Anglicanism

The Archbishop of Canterbury is the head of the Church of England. The religious tradition of the Church of England has contributed most to the culture of Britain and its former colonies. It has retained many more Catholic elements than most Protestant Churches and considers itself to be reformed from the Catholic tradition. African Catholics and Anglicans, who are active members of these denominations, practise their faith in the same way as the majority population.

Islam

According to Giddens (2006) Islam is currently the second largest religion in the world and it is one of the major religions of Africa. Muslims, as adherents of Islam, pray to Allah and Mohammed is his prophet. Muslims attend the local mosque. The basis of Islam is contained in the holy book – the Qur'an.

Five pillars of Islam are:

- belief in Allah, and his prophet Mohammed,
- praying five times a day,
- fasting during the holy month of Ramadan,
- giving of alms to the poor,
- pilgrimage to Mecca, at least once during one's lifetime.

For Muslims the Qur'an is a book of recitation and healing. The Qur'an's purpose is guidance with an emphasis on humanity, its welfare, doing good deeds and to cooperate with all in security and peace (Siddiqui 2008).

Religion and social care

In the UK, there is a historical tradition of religious and faith based agencies providing social welfare and these agencies have had an influence on modern social work (Beckett and Maynard 2005). Child welfare agencies like the welfare charity Barnardo and the Children's Society continue to share their Christian values through discourse and the way in which child welfare services are organized and delivered (Cree 1995). Other social care charities founded by Christians include Samaritans, Shelter, Shaftesbury Society and YMCA (Sentamu 2008). Influenced by care values, practitioners ought to be able to work with religious African families given their adherence to the teachings of their chosen faith. Christian and Islamic teachings subscribe to the core values of caring for humanity. These sit comfortably alongside professional social care principles. This is evidenced through collaborative learning arrangements between universities and the agencies that provide learning opportunities for social care students through practise placements. Statutory social care agencies also work collaboratively with faith based welfare agencies and have in place mechanisms for interagency working with a variety of voluntary sector organizations within the framework of a mixed economy of welfare. Therefore, reaching out to African communities would be in line with current thinking on active service user involvement during planning, delivering, monitoring and evaluating social care services.

Social care management practice

Since religion plays a significant role in the lives of many African families, social care managers could utilize the existing mechanisms for interagency working to ensure that practitioners undertake outreach work through the African church communities as part of their allocated workload and not as additional other. This is important that such activity should not be seen as additional other because, in doing so, it may not be considered essential and, therefore, may not be given the attention it deserves. Appropriate attention is necessary in order to effect change.

In busy social care organizations, practitioners do prioritize essential work. When a decision is taken to engage African faith groups through outreach activities, the mechanism would need to take into account power issues between the two stakeholders – social care statutory service and the African faith group. Social care managers have power and therefore have the ability to influence others to attain desired outcomes. In this case, the influence would focus on ensuring that the practitioners they manage engage in the African community. The process of influence can rely on managers utilizing a mixture of power bases to move things forward in getting social care staff to think outside the routine 'box', and to consider alternative ways of engaging service user groups that they know the least. Engaging African community groups in a meaningful way is important because not enough is known about African family lifestyles and child rearing practices (Olusanya and Hodes 2000). Engaging the wider African community would minimize the chances of making negative assumptions about African families living in the UK.

The mixture of power bases that are commonly cited in literature and worth some consideration here include personal, expert, resource and position power (Huczynski 2004).

Personal power

Personal power is what the individual managers and social care workers bring to the job. This power is the result of the total package of attributes and the impact those attributes have on other people. The attributes of manner, style and personality would be significant because they support the process of influencing others. Used appropriately personal power can demonstrate how a social care practitioner is considerate to others, shows concern for their needs and feelings and treats them fairly and defends their interests. Acknowledging this form of power would be a useful starting point because without analysis practitioners may not fully appreciate their privileged position. By analysing and acknowledging their powerful position, practitioners would find it easier to accomplish a great deal more than they would if they did not fully utilize their position power.

Expert power

This power is based on the expertise held by individuals and the demand for this expertise. The power and influence that stems from highly prized expertise is dependent upon the volume and nature of demand, the location of the expert and their willingness to use the required skills. Expertise could be professional knowledge, technical skills, aptitude and behaviour of social care managers and practitioners.

Resource power

This is a subset of position power. Drawing on this power base enables individuals to exercise authority over the use and allocation of resources. Power over the allocation of resources gives direct power over the activities and the developments that can take place. Resources can be anything that people need and want; therefore, such resources can be used to make things happen. Time is an important resource in social care. Without practitioners giving of their paid time, engagement with those Africans wanting to use social care services would not happen. However, when used appropriately practitioners can make a real difference in people's lives.

Position power

This power is vested in an individual by virtue of their role or position in an organization. It is a form of entitlement. Position power is the main source of authority in organizations and society at large. In social care organizations, position power gives individual managers and practitioners, authority over situations. It entitles individuals to ask questions or to seek information. Huczynski (2004) argues that the greater the range of power bases available to an individual, the greater the choice of strategies that an individual can use. The range highlighted above can be put to good effect in the interest of the group under consideration. Using practitioner power to make things happen in terms of engaging the African community is what this discussion is about, because there has been criticism levelled at statutory social care provision as inappropriate due to tokenistic service user involvement. Power relations lie at the heart of the criticism.

Power issues underlie the majority of identified difficulties with effective user-led change. User participation initiatives require continual awareness of the context of power relations in which they are conducted. Exclusionary structures, institutional practices and professional attitudes can still affect the extent to which service user can influence change.

(SCIE 2004:vii)

By drawing on power base theory to analyse who has the ability to influence others internally and externally can inform positive working relationships in the interest of the service user. Here, I am proposing that a workable partnership is possible between the statutory social care service and the African church based voluntary sector in meeting some of the social care needs of this community. By recognizing and acknowledging the power vested in individual members of each stakeholder group, appropriate services can be developed and delivered.

Example

There is a need to increase the number of foster carers from African communities because African children are overrepresented in local authority care systems. The problem is that community members do not have the knowledge about the workings of social care systems of support for foster carers. Sharing of information about service requirements and the support available to foster carers to enable African community members to gain knowledge would be important. The information sharing process needs to involve existing black foster carers to give first hand accounts of job requirements to community groups, whose members may not be aware that there are African children in the care system, and would benefit from being placed within an African foster family.

To make this change happen, care managers can draw on their power bases and ask for the support they need to reach out to the African community in a targeted way. Central government is keen on user involvement: 'parents, carers and families are the most important influence on outcomes for children and young people' (www.everychildmatters.gov.uk 2008). African families, just like other families will have child rearing expertise that would benefit children in care. Once a decision is taken to work in partnership with African church based groups, it is important to avoid tokenism, because the community in question will lose trust and walk away and the outcomes for African children may be negatively affected. The partnership need not be restricted to church based African community groups. There are other well established African community groups that could be involved if there is a willingness from the statutory sector to share power in a meaningful way. Some critics question the willingness to relinquish and/or share power. Beneath the philosophies and aspirations of handing over power and recognizing people as experts about their own lives who can competently comment on services, lurk the dangers of tokenism (Seden and Ross 2007:199). So, genuine community involvement is strongly recommended in this childcare example, to improve the pool of African foster carers.

The argument in favour of actively engaging the African community in finding effective ways to work with African children is based on the concerns that the existing culture and structure of social care organizations have resulted in the overrepresentation of African children in local authority care. Concerns have been expressed about lack of knowledge on the specificities relating to the care needs of African children at a time when social care practitioners are working to the Every Child Matters agenda. This agenda sets out five priority outcomes for children, which guide service plans. These five priority outcomes are:

- be healthy,
- stay safe,
- enjoy and achieve,
- make a positive contribution,
- achieve economic well-being.

In an effort to achieve these outcomes for African children, it is essential that proactive steps are taken to try alternative ways of working with African families.

Overall, there need not be negative destructive conflict between the values and ethics that inform social care practices and African religious beliefs as discussed earlier. If conflict arises it would need to be acknowledged, managed and confirm areas where the values are complementary in order that progress can be made towards the desired outcomes. Where core values diverge between stakeholders, conflict management would need to rely on the law to support the creation of appropriate and workable strategies. Some African community groups are church based, and others are not, but faith based or not, they both have expertise in welfare issues of importance to Africans across the age range spectrum and as such they have remained an untapped resource. From a practical point of view it would be beneficial for social care practitioners and African community groups to work together as stakeholders with a common goal – that of making a difference in the life of others.

Summary

This chapter has provided insights into:

- African religions,
- the historical significance of religion in colonial Africa,

- the importance of religion among African families in the UK,
- how statutory and voluntary sector partnership working could benefit service users.

Exercise

1   What are the major religions found in Africa south of the Sahara?
2   Why is religious observance prominent in African communities in the UK?
3   How can social care practitioners involve African church groups in welfare work?

9   Ageing, mortality and death

This chapter will:

- discuss the meaning of ageing,
- discuss the ideas about death,
- explore possible practice implications.

Ageing is an inevitable part of life. Culturally, different communities vary in their attitudes to older people. Africans generally respect their elders as people who have become knowledgeable and wise through their life course. In hierarchical terms, older people are placed at the top of the 'tree'. In Africa south of the Sahara, life expectancy is much lower than it is in the West, therefore the numbers of people reaching the age of sixty-five and over is estimated to be around 6 per cent. However, this population is projected to increase to 12 per cent by year 2025. This increase will present some challenges for families because they provide social security to their older members.

Traditionally older people formed an integral part of the fabric of societies across Africa. They played an important role in harmonizing relations when disruptions occurred due to poverty, war and conflict. The complex extended family system has been helpful in enabling effective intergeneration care. Each member within extended family systems, including older members, not only receives, but gives care and advice in return. Under such arrangements older people do not feel redundant or excluded. However, the emerging reality is that Africa is changing with an accelerated pace of urbanization. It is projected that 50 per cent of the African population will be living in towns and cities by year 2020 (Harden 1991). The predictions will divide families into two camps, urban young and rural old. Opinions differ on the sustainability of the extended family system as a force for social security in old age as the following statement illustrates: 'young people, having attended school and secured jobs in cities, find less and less value in the authority, knowledge, and skills of their elders' (Harden 1991:68). However, others consider the isolation of older people in rural Africa as alarmist. Apt (2002) suggests that the emotional ties and economic support among family members remain relatively strong and this is likely to continue for the foreseeable future. Industrialization taking place in Africa is affecting the traditional care systems organized around the family resulting in possible reduction in harmonious existence, young people seek paid work away from their rural environments and cost implications of maintaining urban and rural homes on limited income.

Poverty is a major concern, particularly among widows (Owen 1996). Marriage patterns, with specific reference to polygamy, expose widows to real hardship and marginalization. To reduce the levels of poverty and lack of employment opportunities, international migration in search of employment and better prospects has been a significant feature among Africans since the 1980s. International migration and loss of sons to war and HIV/AIDS has meant that older relations are left behind without money or the traditional support network. Some of the widows have faired well through international migration to the West and have been able to send remittances back home meeting their obligations towards their older relatives dependent on them for welfare. The inevitability of ageing is catching up with the African migrants who came to the UK perhaps with a view to make their fortune then return to their country of origin. The reality is that the majority have not managed to save any money let alone accumulating a financial fortune, and are now facing the prospect of growing old in the UK, and are considering their retirement. Can they afford to retire? Will the financial poverty they left in Africa catch up with them? Where is the final resting place when they die? These are some of the questions to which African older people are likely to want to find answers. Social care workers who come into contact with African older people could have a dialogue based on these questions with a view to working with them towards identifying solutions.

Literature on ethnicity and old age is limited for obvious reasons of comparative youth. Minority adults who came to the UK during the 1960s and 1970s are now senior citizens and, as such, there are signs that ethnicity will be taken into account in future social policy research on old age. Research studies that are shaping the knowledge base on ageing and social care have confirmed some similarity as well as differences, for example on issues of informal care.

> A clear finding from this study is that in terms of their descriptions of the experience of informal care, South Asians and African Caribbean family members appear to experience caring in largely the same way as that of which has been in the large literature on informal care based on the majority population.
>
> (Adamson and Donovan 2005:47)

Such similarities are echoed in the study by Moriarty and Butt (2004) on the quality of life among older people from minority communities and state that the majority of participants across all ethnic groups attached considerable importance to their relationships with members of their family and friends in contributing to their quality of life. Additionally, Gabriel and Bowling (2004) also found that the central planks of quality of life among older people were social relationships, home and neighbourhood social capital, health and functional ability and social roles and activities. The evidence from the various studies has implications for African families who provide informal care to a small but growing population of their older people living in the UK, currently estimated to be around 2 per cent of the total African population. While this figure is significantly lower than the equivalent age group in Africa south of the Sahara, estimated to be about 6 per cent, such a manageable size of the population provides a window of opportunity to work with African community groups to ensure that those aspects of social care that are specific to this particular group are adequately addressed. Planning for the development of appropriate and sensitive provision is necessary because the deficit in service provision to older people from ethnic minority communities has long been recognized (Department of Health 2002b, Social Services Inspectorate 2002, Ahmad 1990).

Poverty has been highlighted as an issue of concern among some pensioners because they make up a disproportionate share of those with the lowest income (Llewellyn *et al.* 2008). The employment patterns of African immigrants and their earning capacity would suggest a likelihood of living on low incomes – mainly state pension in retirement. Pension poverty has specific significance for African older people because of extended family dependants in Africa. These pensioners may be poor by UK standards, but unfortunately their kin continue to expect to receive remittances to enable them to survive the harsh conditions linked to abject poverty. The felt need to offer financial support to the extended family back in African remains strong. It is what most Africans still feel obligated to do and, as such, it needs to be acknowledged because of possible implications for the psychological well-being of this group of older people, with interests in two camps.

The pressure to continue to provide financial support to extended family members back in Africa was articulated by all the participants in the survey of social work students and practising social workers, suggesting that it is an important issue they must address, as well as those who work with African families. Meeting the needs of the immediate family in the UK can be compromised by spreading limited resources thinly in order to accommodate, also, the needs of kith and kin back in Africa. Because of these responsibilities and interests among older people in particular specific attention would be necessary. Their vulnerabilities would need to be assessed taking into account their life histories including patterns of migration and how they have managed their integration in mainstream society.

Schroder-Butterfill and Marianti's (2006) systematic framework for approaching vulnerability in old age using constituent domains of exposure, threats, coping capacities and outcomes could usefully be considered, given that the impact of migration on old age can be linked to education, geographical location, housing and employment histories (Alcock 1997). The majority of Africans have tended to settle in inner city deprived areas of the UK, as highlighted in Chapter 1. A variety of reasons are well documented (Equality Review 2007, Evans *et al.* 2005, Daley 1998). Some of the reasons discussed in the studies include newness, limited knowledge of the labour market and racial discrimination, which forced some to take low paid jobs, thereby compounding the cycle of deprivation. The strong family ties with those that remained in Africa and the financial support that is maintained possibly affected their ability to move away from deprived areas in preparation for their retirement. However, for this group of older people there are benefits to be had by remaining within established African communities in major cities as discussed in Chapter 1. African older people can be less isolated as they continue to associate with other Africans in places of worship and attendance at cultural events. The nature and extent of vulnerability can be assessed using a framework aid that examines the interactions among the domains of exposure, threats, coping capacities and outcomes (Schroder and Marianti 2006).

Participants to the survey question about ageing and mortality yielded results to suggest that, for some, their thought processes remain firmly connected with Africa but, for others, living for the moment was considered to be important. These differences have implications for individual life histories. For example, those who retain the expectation of social care within the family, group care living in care homes is likely to be alien among these Africans. This concern is probably due to the fact that these Africans, throughout their working lives, would have maintained their connection with an African approach to providing care for their older people. Internalization of this traditional African norm as the best way of looking after older people while residing away from Africa makes it difficult for some to make the transition towards accepting a UK norm of some provision of group care living towards the end of life. Expectations to be cared for by their children in old age remain very strong, as indicated by the survey participants, while acknowledging that the practicalities of living arrangements in the UK can make such expectations unrealistic. Such expectations may have been reinforced by exposure to the vulnerability of older people in group care homes leading them towards a decision that the African way is a better option. If this unrealistic expectation is to be addressed social care policy has a part to play. With regards to the issues surrounding preparation for end of life and death, the importance of community support was indicated to be significant, particularly during the bereavement period. For those who have retained African customs and traditions on dying and death, the ceremonies can be elaborate and expensive. According to survey participants, the body of the deceased and its soul needs special care as well as providing gender specific emotional support to the bereaved. Repatriation of the dead to their country of origin is a common practice among Africans. Custom requires that gifts of money are presented to the bereaved family to help defray funeral expenses. For example, among the Shona people of Zimbabwe, this financial gift is known as *chema* and each person attending the home of the bereaved would be expected to contribute what they can: there is no set figure.

Arrangements for repatriating the dead to Africa would not be possible for many Africans who wish to be buried in their country of origin without voluntary financial donation from community group members. Participants pointed out that a recognition of poverty within UK based African communities has influenced the creation of self-help societies in line with a long-standing tradition in many African countries. In these countries there is a tradition going back many years, of establishing religious societies, saving groups and burial societies (Kaseke 1999).

These traditions are now replicated in the UK, to minimize hardships at the time of death as previously stated. Interconnectedness and community involvement as key features of family life in Africa south of the Sahara, appear to influence the way in which the participants considered end of life issues. Their considerations are reflected in Karenga's (1993) analysis of African traditional religions and concluded that the religions have influenced cultural practices that remain prevalent at home and abroad. Death is seen as another stage in human development, and that humans are born, live, die and become the ancestors, thus death is not the end, but the beginning of another form of existence. He suggests that the idea of ancestral spirits is linked to personal and collective immortality. Africans who select their country of origin as their final resting place would suggest that their decisions might be informed by African religious traditions even though they may be practising Christians. Perhaps this can be seen as the Africanization of Christianity, an infusion of the two religions. The following statements provide insights into the views of the majority of the survey participants about the end of life among Africans post-migration and settlement. 'Most migrants dread the concept of living in care homes and prefer instead to be able to make provisions for old age back in Africa unless their children are able to care for them at home' (student social worker-participant (2)).

> Older African people living in the UK believe that there is life after this life, that death is not the end of us. This belief helps them deal with mortality. Death is accepted as part of life. Death itself does not scare them. I think having a healthy appreciation for mortality can help them appreciate each day and the beauty around them. It is some what comforting to know that they have a final resting place waiting for them, but really it is more important that they live their life to the fullest and be remembered for it.
>
> (Practising social worker: participant (10))

For most of the communities, there exists the support net-work of compatriots, which often try to give a resemblance of what would be the case in the native country. Older folk usually understand that the busy life here, leave little time and room for extended bereavement and grief.

(Practising social worker: participant (25))

Africans believe that their final resting place is their home town or village in Africa. Many make arrangement/plans about their bodies being flown back to Africa when they die. They believe their bodies should not be buried in a foreign land (UK) because their souls would be lost.

(Student social worker: participant (23))

We still fly our dead back home than bury them here. We believe that one member of the family buried here will be a lost soul, so the dead must be taken home to be among the souls of other deceased family members.

(Student social worker: participant (13))

Grief within a cultural context and practical support are encapsulated in this statement:

This varies from one group to another, but there are overwhelming similarities in terms of grieving. It takes the form of crying out loud, singing songs of praise, retelling achievements and relying on close friends and relatives to seek solace. Also paying homage/respect to the deceased is equally significant. It is almost obligatory among friends and acquaintances to visit the deceased's family to comfort and grieve with them as this helps to lubricate and promote community spirit and to deal with loss. Making a financial contribution plays a vital role to help with funeral arrangements. The visits from friends and sundry provisions usually last until the funeral right is complete, as a way of reassuring family members and to reduce isolation. Within our community (Sierra Leone), the women normally volunteer and take turns to prepare meals and to welcome visitors. This takes away the burden from immediate family members. The frenzied flow of sympathizers helps minimise the impact and foster cohesion among us.

(Practising social worker: participant (17))

Nangoli (1986) articulated similar sentiments highlighted by participant (17) in relation to the interactions that are expected, the grieving process that involves wailing, singing story telling and specific roles played by men and women.

It can therefore be said that within African communities in the UK, bereavement is not individualized, it is a community affair, particularly among the older generation who expect at least more than a few days of communal support. This is particularly important among those Africans who came to the UK and belong to a generation of people with cultural ties to Africa that have remained strong. Culture in this sense would be reflected in languages they speak, the way they behave, live, relate to one another, worship their God, regard their children, treat older people, bury the dead and generally conduct themselves in a way that distinguishes them from people of the world who are not black Africans. Unfortunately, research evidence, specific to the way in which Africans resident in the UK deal with death and bereavement, is not available. Until such a time when empirical evidence becomes available, social care practitioners working with bereaved Africans would need to accept the challenge of being guided by individual families and their communities about their specific practices and rituals. In this case, acknowledging limitations should be seen as a weakness, but appreciate a strength that can be tapped into as part of a learning process to acquire new knowledge.

Currer (2007:47) reminds social workers about the importance of not making assumptions, and states, when you are working with someone who is visibly different from yourself, because they are from a different cultural or racial background, you may be alerted to the impact of social issues. Yet these are important to all of us, and we should not assume that we share a common view without checking this out.

Checking things out with African families is equally important in view of the diversity that is inherent within African cultural practices. In their study on older people's views about home as a place of care and end of life, Gott *et al.* (2004) found that the views expressed were varied but concluded that older people wanted choice between hospital and palliative care at home. Facilitating choice would be beneficial to Africans who may have difficulty in accepting institutional care. For some of these Africans, the concept of home may be their African home town or village.

Summary

This chapter has provided insights into:

- views about ageing among Africans,
- views about the way Africans deal with dying and death,
- views about bereavement, the grieving process and burial.

Exercise

1   What is the nature of support available to African older people?
2   How do most Africans express their grief?
3   Why do some African people wish to be buried in their countries of origin?

10 Negotiating and balancing the demands from two cultures

This chapter will:

- discuss issues of cultural identity,
- discuss issues of integration,
- explore coping strategies.

Identity

According to Ruth (2006), identity is about who we are and what we are. For Africans as the group under consideration, they will have a range of different social or cultural identities. These multiple identities play a part in shaping the way they think, feel and act. Ruth goes on to suggest that identities can be categorized into specific labels such as colour, religion, gender and age. However, it needs to be acknowledged that the categories listed do not represent an exhaustive list, because there are many more categories people can identify with. For each individual, some of these identities will be more significant than others. The enduring identities can be grouped under the social category umbrella (Nkomo and Cox 1996). These broader social categories are likely to be more salient for most people, but this should not be taken for granted. However, identities that are significant play a stronger role than less significant ones in shaping the way people are in terms of the values and priorities that people attach to their lives (Ruth 2006). He goes on to suggest that key identities vary from time to time during people's lifetime due to ever changing situations that bring about greater awareness of self. It seems therefore relevant that individuals regularly reflect on their key identities that make them who they are, as a basis for maintaining a positive self-image. This positive self-image can be promoted through cultural identity resulting from shared history and ancestry that an identifiable group of people hold in common. Hall (1990) considers that cultural identities are important because they reflect historical experiences and cultural codes which provide people with a frame of reference. This frame of reference enables people to move back and forth because cultural identity belongs to the future as well as to the past, suggesting that cultural identities undergo constant transformation. Cultural identity of Africans in the twenty-first century has been shaped by a shared history and ancestry as well as the shared experience of being colonized by a people with a different history. On migration to the West, Africans would rely of their cultural identity as frame of reference to assist them in negotiating a successful path in a foreign land. In view of this, it would seem appropriate to raise a generic question on issues of identity.

How do Africans living in the UK see themselves? Based on Elam and Chinouya's (2000) study on African populations living in the UK, a number of factors were found to be significant in people's identities: age, immigration status, nationality and country of origin. Older and younger people identified with Africa in divergent ways; strong connection with Africa was noted as significant among older people and less among younger people, who identified more readily with European culture. Exclusion from opportunities to secure British citizenship was found to have contributed to externalization, thereby creating an identity of the 'other'. In view of the differences of identity between older and younger people, both groups would need to deal with issues of identity, but in different ways, particularly if there are internalized negativities resulting from life experiences. It is necessary that African families living in the UK deal with issues of identity: a number of studies have indicated that there are correlations between negative racial identity and low self-esteem (Lester 2000, Maxime 1993, Cross 1980, 1991). The techniques used to address issues of low self-esteem associated with racial identity would need to be age specific because young people and adults will have different histories to tell. Apart from age considerations in planning intervention methods, parental backgrounds would need to be taken into account because some people may have one parent who is black African and the other who is white European. This group of people with a dual heritage has received research attention and exercised the minds of social care workers. In view of this, attention is needed to address identity issues specific to them with a view to learn about best practices and isolating areas for future research. Currently there are young people, whose parents are African and European, and therefore have a dual heritage. In discussing African family life, it is important to take into account the views of children with a mixed cultural identity. There are polarized ideological debates in academic circles about identity issues and mixed families. One camp favours a black perspective for all children of African and European heritage, the other camp preferring a mixed perspective (Barn and Harman 2006). This polarization suggests that the politics of race and ethnicity is still exercising the minds of many who have an interest or work in the field of social care. Perhaps the solution need not be that complicated because it lies within the individual. Therefore, listening to young people about self-categorization with the support of their parents would seem to be appropriate. Research evidence suggests that many categorize themselves as having two cultural identities that they tap into to produce a new one (Caballero *et al.* 2008).

For some young people in the UK, they find their own way of dealing with demands from two cultures such that their self-esteem is not affected. For others the situation may be different and conflict can arise within families. Sometimes such families do come to the attention of external agencies such as those that provide statutory or voluntary social care support. Reasons for conflict can be associated with different values between generations in terms of accepted social behaviour among the young as illustrated by the following statement.

> While some adolescents have arrived from overseas, others are the children of first, or second generation immigrants or belong to minority groups who have been in the UK over hundreds of years. Their values and expectations, or that of their families, may be different from those of the majority community, particularly on issues concerning social behaviour, sexual relationships and marriage, and educational and career choices.
>
> (Taylor 2003:52)

In dealing with these differences that cause conflict within families Taylor (2003) suggests that practitioners who work with black adolescents may consider the use of Sue *et al.*'s (1998) minority identity development model (MID) that follows a five stage process, because it is thought that the model is usable among a variety of minority groups whose children find themselves growing up within a different majority culture. It is recommended as a tool that can be used among others. Another approach for consideration is Cross's (1980) black identity nigrescence model. The focus of this model is a four stage process of becoming black among those people who hold a Eurocentric worldview. This model is considered to be useful as it enables people to understand problems of black identity confusion. The model also provides material to support an examination of what happens to a person during identity change or transformation since identity attitudes are not fixed (Robinson 2000). The stages of each model are described below.

Minority identity development model

Minority identity developmental model can be used to explore the various stages that are likely to be experienced by minority young people of African descent as they develop a new cultural identity. The model describes the five stages of the process that an immigrant African child might go through starting with childhood.

Stage one: conformity

The African immigrant children prefer the dominant majority group's cultural values and norms such as birthday parties, sleepovers and food and meal preparation. They may denigrate their own culture. They will do so because they want to be part of the group and, therefore, conform and see themselves as members of the majority culture. The way they behave and generally conduct themselves would be reflective of the majority culture.

Stage two: dissonance

The pressure from home and peers slowly causes the individual African child to break down. The pressure penetrates the denial wall and the child begins to accept that they are 'different'. The acceptance of difference leads the child to become aware of the positive aspects and strengths of their African values and norms. The awareness brings with it feelings of shame and embarrassment about their previously held conformity attitudes.

Stage three: resistance and immersion

The individual begins to appreciate and endorse only their own African minority group's strengths. They may go out of their way to be seen to vehemently reject white middle-class cultural norms. The wearing of dreadlocks among African young people can be an example to demonstrate resistance and non-conformity.

Stage four: introspection

The questioning continues as the African young person begins to question their own rigidly held views and cultural practices. They increasingly turn their attention to themselves as an individual and begin to value their autonomy.

Stage five: synergetic articulation and awareness

The individual begins to find a psychologically healthy balance between their belonging to their own African minority group and their comfortable participation in the wider majority culture. They feel self-fulfilment in regard to their own African cultural identity and increasingly self-confident about all their cross-cultural relationships in the adult world. However, evidence suggests that it may be difficult for the young person to engage in stages four and five when they are still living in the parental home. However, practitioners working with African young people could use this model to assist them in considering the stage the individual may have reached. To do this, the process could include direct observation of the young person's behaviour and attitude towards:

- members of their own African cultural group,
- members of another minority cultural group,

- members of the majority cultural group,
- themselves.

The results of the observations could then be used to inform the nature of intervention (adapted from Taylor 2003:56).

Black identity negrescience model

This is a four stage process of transformation, from pre-encounter to internalization. The theoretical tool can be used to illuminate understanding of the potential dynamic of identity negotiation.

Stage one: pre-encounter (or pre-discovery)

The African person is considered to be out of touch with herself or himself racially and the person's worldview is dominated by European determinants. They subscribe to a white normative standard; the end result at this stage of the process is pro-white and anti-black.

Stage two: encounter (or discovery)

A shocking personal or social event pushes an African person past her or his conceptions of black and black conditions. Their receptiveness to new views of being black in the world leads to intense search for black identity.

Stage three: immersion/emersion

It is a period of transition in which an African person struggles to destroy all vestiges of the old perspectives and immerse into total blackness and withdraw from interaction with white people. This withdrawal phase is followed by a levelling off from the oversimplified aspects of blackness leading to an acceptance of white humanity.

Stage four: internalization/commitment

It is a phase in which an African person becomes less defensive, achieves inner security, has self-confidence with blackness and uses black people as a primary reference group. The new confidence enables the individual to move towards adopting a pluralistic non-racist perspective (adapted from Robinson 2000, Karenga 1993).

The two models, minority development model and negrescience model, can be considered for possible use in supporting practitioners in search of theories that can help them analyse the complexities associated with cultural identity among African young people resident in the UK. What is important is that criticality is not compromised; therefore, practitioners who select to use these two theoretical models should do so cautiously, especially when supporting young people with self-esteem issues.

It is argued that establishing cultural identity is fraught with difficulties, and as such young people negotiating two cultures need support from significant adults. Cultural identity has implications for self-esteem, self-concept and emotional development (Paludi 2002, Moghaddam 1998). For African families living in the UK, as with other ethnic minority families, it is important to establish their methods of support to their children to enable young people to effectively manage the demands from two cultures. With the support of their African community, their social care practitioner, a young person can be well placed to determine how best to integrate.

Survey results suggested that this was an area that many African parents find to be the most challenging, suggesting that cultural identity issues have not been sorted. In summary, participants concurred that this was the most challenging area for most African families, regardless of their reasons for migrating to the UK. Issues specific to children were repeatedly singled out in that the nature of support from within the family depended on cultural values in relation to language spoken at home, food and diet, social behaviour and dealing with peer pressure. The importance of supporting children was fully acknowledged and it seems that most parents work hard at this, even though there was a sense they seldom get it right. Concerns were expressed as to whether parents should seek professional help when the 'going gets tough' and when they do, how will they be perceived? Selected statements provide a summary of the approaches used by parents to include:

> Some Africans do this by taking their children back to their countries of origin for holidays so as to present to them both cultures. As much as possible prepare and eat African food as they would back home and teach them the parents' first language. They get the children involved in as many African cultural activities as possible when they are still young. They talk to their children about the two cultures and help them to choose good practices from both. This remains a challenge. While there is a lot of talk about encouraging children to remain true to their roots, work culture dictates that there is insufficient time to counteract new influences and to spend time together as a family or even visiting family and friends.

One participant encapsulated the views of the majority and stated balancing the demands from the two cultures is an area where most African families find to be extremely challenging. Perhaps it is quite easy to those who have young children, but quite hard when they are teenagers. Most families try to maintain their cultural values at home by speaking their languages, eating their traditional food and attending cultural events as families but as the children get older, they just want to be like their white peers and yet their identity is not white.

To summarize, the views expressed by the majority of the participants can be categorized into the following themes:

- modelling
- African holidays
- education through ongoing dialogue
- bilingualism
- availability
- advice.

Given the overrepresentation of African children in care, corporate parenting of African children by local authorities would need to emulate the themes highlighted above in order to achieve the positive outcomes as stipulated by the Every Child Matters agenda. The incorporation of African parenting styles on cultural identity issues can involve engagement with communities with training input and research. The extent to which these approaches produce the desired outcomes have only been assessed by African communities and individual families, and African people share tips and techniques among themselves as best as they can, through church attendance, community group functions and among friends. What is in the public domain are the problem areas and an overrepresentation in terms of the numbers of African children that have been received into local authority care, and concerns about the quality of care the children receive (Bernard and Gupta 2008). Additionally, what is also known by the public at large is generally through the media whose attention tend to focus on the negative aspects and social work obligations to supporting those in need. With regard to children in need, Graham (2002) offers a view that social work often deals with children in difficult situations and circumstances, away from their families and environments, yet we know very little about children's own interpretation or understanding of these experiences. African community involvement can make a contribution to this. It can be argued that if African parenting practices are not fully understood, it is likely that African children in care and who are not given the opportunity to articulate their understanding of their life experiences, can become even more confused about their identity and how to relate to their families when they become reunited. In addition to trialling identity theoretical models when undertaking one to one work with African young people in care it is important to use community expertise as well as giving a voice to each young person along the lines suggested by Graham (2007).

Some ideas for consideration

Graham (2007), in her article about giving a voice to black children, provides a useful framework as illustrated below.

- The emphasis is on acknowledging bicultural competence, enabling the children to speak and be heard.
- Acknowledging impact of poverty and contributory structural factors and take remedial action and make appropriate resources available.
- Avoidance of family pathologies and emulating successful African family parenting practices, established through engaging African communities.
- Actively involve African communities in child welfare research, and in finding solutions to presenting problems.
- Utilize the Every Child Matters Agenda to address the needs of African children and their families.

Despite the experience of racism and discrimination, there are African families living in the UK who are successfully managing to help their children to make meaningful and healthy transitions into the British way of life. It is from the experiences of these families that a great deal more can be learnt. Empirical evidence on what works and is cost effective is long overdue.

Summary

This chapter has provided insights into:

- methods used by Africans to support children through cultural change,
- identity issues and suggested theoretical identity models for potential use,
- a framework for supporting families in a meaningful way.

Case study

Fafi is a fourteen year old African child. She arrived in the UK to join her parents when she was ten. She had been left in the care of her maternal aunt in the country of origin for a period of two years, while she attended boarding school during term time. On arrival in the UK, she continued with her education and attended the local school. Fafi settled into her new environment reasonably well, but repeatedly told her parents that she missed her friends back home in Africa. By the age of thirteen tensions were growing between Fafi and her parents because she wanted to go out for leisure with her school friends most evenings. She frequently told her parents that she hated the African way of life because it was backward and wished she lived with her white friend's family. Ongoing tension within the family was resulting in frequent outbursts on both sides – parents and child. Fafi's mother, without consulting her husband, decided that the family needed help, so she visited her local social services department to ask for help.

1   What might be the reasons for the projected behaviours?
2   How would you assess the needs of this family?
3   Discuss your answers with your peers.

Conclusion

This chapter will:

- summarize the main points from all the chapters,
- highlight specific practice issues,
- offer a framework for change.

Reflecting back to my attempt to convey a particular message about social care with African families is the focus of this chapter. The process involved the use of literature and empirical evidence to support the discussion on issues singled out to be of importance to an understanding of African family life. Materials are organized into ten chapter segments and the main points to emerge from the discussion are included in this chapter. The message throughout has been about changing the way Africans are perceived by those who provide and deliver social care services with a view to encouraging practitioners to consider alternative approaches to working with African families. A framework for working with change is included in this chapter.

Chapter 1 provided contextual information about Africans living in the region south of the Sahara desert, paying attention to size and population characteristics, state of economic development and international media portrayal of the African continent and its people. This information was linked to issues of migration to illustrate the journey's end to the UK and the lived experiences of Africans in their adopted country. Social care issues of concern to and about Africans living in the UK were discussed, and included poverty, employment, education, mental health and the over-representation of African children in the statutory social care system. Suggestions were put forward to tackle the difficulties and problems faced by African families.

Chapters 2 and 3 are closely related in that they sought to provide a policy context in which social care is operationalized. Social welfare provision and the ideological drivers were discussed, together with the management and leadership structures in place to make things happen for the group under consideration. At government policy level, ideas about citizenship and entitlement to welfare support were noted to be a drawback and impacted on organizational structures that service the welfare state, resulting in some poor Africans being excluded from receiving appropriate support.

The thinking around the writing of this book stemmed from a positive response to a questionnaire I circulated to past and present African social work students at the University of Reading about social care with African families. Chapter 4 highlighted key findings and these provided the structure to the remainder of the chapters. Racism and discrimination featured in most of their responses, but they saw a way out of the impasse, and this was very encouraging.

Discussion in Chapter 5 considered education and employment issues based on the views of survey participants about the experiences of African people and the way they cope with the pressures they encounter. The pressures were found to be linked to poverty and race based exclusion from opportunities that are accessible to the rest of the population. Constant rejection led some to internalize the oppression, thereby perpetuating a vicious cycle of exclusion and adding more pressure on African family life. Having considered the pressures experienced by families, the discussion moved attention to the specifics and nature of African family life. In Chapter 6, marriage systems were explained with a particular emphasis on bride-price and the payment of bride-wealth that remains common among Africans at home and abroad. The advantages and disadvantages of this tradition between women and men were noted. In addition to bride-wealth, another tradition that has stood the taste of time is the prevalence of polygamous marriages throughout the continent of Africa south of the Sahara. Christians, African feminists and national gender equality laws are influencing debates towards changing these marriage systems. The evidence suggests that for now polygamous marriages and the payment of bride-wealth are part of African family life.

Chapter 7 identified family patterns and child rearing practices that were considered to be common among Africans. The extended family was noted to be a norm and that child rearing was confirmed to be the responsibility of this extended family network. This arrangement has benefits in supporting working parents with free childcare. In relation to Africans living in the UK, community and faith groups were identified to be playing a useful role in replicating the African tradition of communal care for young children. African children are expected to show respect to their elders in culture specific ways, such as bowing, clasping hands together and not to address elders by their names. Discipline is also very important within African families and parents use similar methods to those used by the majority of the population. Interracial marriage patterns were noted to be on the increase and, as a result, the debates in academic circles have focused on issues of cultural identity with regards to mixed race children, given their overrepresentation in the care system.

The discussion in Chapter 8 focused on religion and spirituality based on survey results. The main points to emerge suggested that on the whole, most Africans were considered to be religious and were active participants of their chosen faith. This was demonstrated by regular church attendance. This active involvement influenced their lifestyles. However, their African norms and traditions informed the way in which they practised their religion as Christians or Muslims. This is possibly because both religions as they are known today were introduced to Africa during the period of colonization. Therefore Africans have incorporated aspects of African traditional religion into their current style of worship. Religion and spirituality were closely connected to ideas about mortality and death that are the main focus in Chapter 9. Ageing and dying were just accepted as part of life. No fears were expressed according to the results of the survey. Repatriation of the dead to Africa was seen as imperative to enable the soul to join the ancestors. Community members rally around and provide financial and emotional support to the bereaved in a way that resembles current practice in most African countries south of the Sahara. An extended period of mourning is preferred but societal functions in the UK were acknowledged to be different, therefore adjustments continue to be made within the African community.

Chapter 10 focused on issues of identity in relation to parental support made available to African children who must balance the demands from two cultures. The main issue to note was the acknowledgement from all the survey participants that biculturalism was the most challenging area they grapple with. Various techniques were commonly used such as: bilingualism, open dialogue, role modelling, African holidays and being available to answer questions. In addition, African parents place a great deal of emphasis in providing education about their African culture as well as highlighting the positive aspects of the UK culture to enable their children access to the most helpful aspects in support of their integration and personal well-being. Within this chapter two models are included for consideration when practitioners are planning identity work with African children in the care system.

The insights into the historical background and experiences of Africans shared within the ten chapters of this book seem to suggest that change is necessary in order to improve the lives of African families living in the UK who come into contact with social care practitioners. Directing this change requires effective leadership and management and willingness among practitioners to try something different. Cited in the introduction is a statement from a practising social worker expressing concern that anti-oppressive practice remains aspirational and that management seemed not to care about ineffective and inappropriate interventions afforded to some African families. It is against this backdrop that ideas about managing change are explained. Changing the way social care practitioners interact with African families cannot be ignored because available evidence discussed in Chapter

1 shows that the African population is increasing, and that a significant number of African families live in poverty. They are in poverty due to unemployment and underemployment. Because of this, some families will come to the attention of social services. It is important, therefore, that preventative social care work is undertaken, particularly in the area of child welfare to stop the overrepresentation of African children in local authority care systems. The need to do things differently is encapsulated in the following statement:

> At present, social work in England often falls short of these basic conditions for success. Weakness in recruitment, retention, frontline resources, training, leadership, public understanding and other factors are all compounding one another. They are holding back the profession and making service improvements difficult to achieve. Most importantly, people who look to social workers for support are not getting the consistently high quality of service they deserve.
>
> (Social Work Task Force 2009:9)

Managing change

I would endorse that African families who look to social workers for support have not always received a consistently high quality service and for that reason, I would argue that proactive change is necessary and issues relating to training and leadership are important in order to transform the way practitioners see themselves in relation to their capacity to deliver relevant service to African families. Both transformational and transactional leadership qualities can be relied upon to support the change. This combination is termed transformactional (Champayne *et al.* 2007). It is a term intended to reflect the fact that a transformational leader is able to challenge the status quo and implement change and a transactional leader regularly deliver results without affecting the overall direction of the organization hence, transformactional leadership.

This proactive change is aimed at enabling staff members to understand the need to work with African community groups to gain knowledge about the specificities of African family life. To progress this, leaders and managers need to give attention to the impact the change will have throughout their service area. With that clarity, they can then involve others. Force Field analysis is a useful tool commonly used because it provides a holistic picture of a situation whilst enabling the participant to deal with its component parts in manageable chunks. The analysis can be initially organized into a seven steps sequence as follows:

- define ideal state,
- define worst imaginable state,
- define current state of equilibrium,

- identify restraining forces,
- identify helping forces,
- create a map of helping and restraining forces,
- work out a strategy for reducing restraining forces while maintaining helpful forces and present level.

The selected strategy for reducing restraining forces will enable a movement from steady state to unfreezing to take place. At the steady state staff members feel that change is unnecessary and that their service organization is performing well in delivering services to African communities. By sharing information on deficits and reminding staff members the core values of social care, unfreezing takes place. At this stage practices that stand in the way of change are excluded in order that the movement can happen and staff members begin to think and perform differently. Refreezing takes place when new norms and standards about working with African families are established.

Lewin's (1947) change model summary:

Steady state → unfreezing → changing → refreezing

As with any model, there are limitations in terms of usefulness, but this one has stood the test of time due to its simplicity. It helps people to be clear about what needs to change and why, even if they may not agree with the planned change. By using the tool, the aim is to encourage ownership of the change as something that social care practitioners need in order to meet their job requirements. The focus of the change is about engaging the African community in a new and different way. To lead the change requires imagination, creativity and commitment. Through effective engagement with the African community, social care practitioners will be better placed to receive the key messages articulated by African social work students.

A summarized list of the main messages for social care practitioners is listed below: when interacting with African families social care workers would be expected to continue to be guided by the GSCC codes of practice and adhere to the core values to ensure that they practise in an anti-oppressive way.

African children will not speak up in the presence of relatives and significant adults. So, as part of an assessment, children need to be allowed space to communicate, away from significant adults. This way of working falls within the existing guidelines about hearing children's voices as users of social care services; therefore, it should be the norm for all children and conducted within a cultural context.

Some Africans may see a handshake as a sign of friendship, so be aware! An acknowledgement that many Africans experience racial discrimination and feel oppressed is very important and then support them with coping strategies. Because the UK will be a new experience, there needs to be an appreciation that African families need time to adapt and that parental control is not abuse or neglect. African teenagers often experience cultural pressures from within the home and cultural pressure outside the home as well as racism: do not add any more pressure. There needs to be an appreciation that some African families try to ensure that baby-sitting is arranged amongst themselves. Often church based relationships are considered most reliable, including third party introductions. At times, there might be private fostering/respite arrangements in place for a limited duration for young people having difficulty living with birth parents at home. During this time, there might be informal talks with the young person/ parents, sharing ideas on how to support the situation. This needs to be acknowledged.

The summarized list above sits comfortably alongside the ideas contained in the Audit Commission Report (2004), with an emphasis on a business like approach to managing social care services informed by the values of social care. It is therefore appropriate that social care managers, as part of their leadership role, can be asked to develop services that respond appropriately to the needs of African families, given their lived experience of enduring racism and social exclusion (Oko 2008). In line with current thinking on service user involvement, partnership working and power sharing, it is equally important that the African community comes forward and challenges the status quo, seeks ways for self-empowerment and liberation through allegiances with other minority groups and publicizing positive aspects of African family life. As a final note, it may be useful to refer back to the Introduction and reconsider the question – why this book? For me the answer is connected with wanting to share some information that might be of use to social care students who are likely to come into contact with African families during their period of training. It is important that social care practitioners acknowledge that African families living in the UK brought with them their cultural norms about family life. These norms provide a framework for making sense of the new environment and how to negotiate their way through complex social care systems. They selected to migrate to the UK for a better life and are prepared to work hard to achieve success. However, despite good levels of formal education and professional qualifications, many are underemployed and end up taking more than one job to make ends meet. Actively involving African families in finding solutions to the problems they face is a strategy worthy of serious consideration, in the interest of that well rehearsed value of social justice.

Appendix

Social care with Sub-Saharan African families questionnaire

1 What role do religion, faith and spirituality play among Africans living in the UK?
2 How do older African people living in the UK, deal with mortality, death and final resting place issues?
3 How do African families support their children, balance the demands from two cultures – country of origin and current place of residence?
4 How do Africans living in the UK discipline their children?
5 What are some of the child rearing practices that are familiar to you?
6 How do marriage practices such as bride-price affect structures and power relations within the family?
7 What do you consider to be the main pressures experienced by African families living in the UK in relation to:

   a   employment?
   b   education?

8 What other information not addressed in questions 1–7 do you consider to be important for social care workers to know, in order to support their practice when interacting with African families?

References

Achebe, C. (1960) *No Longer At Ease*. London: Heinemann.

Adair, J. (2002) *Effective Strategic Leadership*. Basingstoke: Palgrave Macmillan.

Adamson, J. Donovan, J. (2005) Normal disruption: South Asian and African/Caribbean relatives caring for an older family member in the UK. *Social Science and Medicine*, Vol. 60, No. 1, pp. 37–48.

Adomako Ampofo, A., Beoku-Betts, J., Njambi, W.N. (2004) Women and gender studies English-speaking Sub-Saharan Africa. *Gender and Society*, Vol. 28, No. 6, pp. 685–714.

African Population and Health Research Centre (2008) Population Data. Nairobi: PRB and APHRC.

AFRUCA (2008) *Promoting the Rights and Welfare of African Children*. London: AFRUCA.

Ahmad, B. (1990) *Black Perspectives in Social Work*. Birmingham: Venture Press.

Alcock, P. (1993) *Understanding Poverty*. Basingstoke: Palgrave Macmillan.

Alcock, P. (1997) *Understanding Poverty* (2nd edn). Basingstoke: Palgrave Macmillan.

Alcock, P. (2003) *Social Policy in Britain*. Basingstoke: Palgrave Macmillan.

Aldgate, J., Healey, L., Malcolm, B., Pine, B., Rose, R., Seden, J. (2007) *Enhancing Social Work Management*. London: Jessica Kingsley.

Amadiume, I. (2000) *Daughters of the Goddess: Daughters of Imperialism*. London: Zed Books.

Andersen, M.L., Hill Collins, P. (1998) *Race Class and Gender*. London: Wadsworth Publishing Company.

Apt, N.A. (2002) Ageing and the changing role of the family and the community: An African perspective. *International Social Security Review*, Vol. 55, No. 1, pp. 39–47.

Audit Commission and Social Services (2004) *Old Virtues, New Virtues*. London: Audit Commission.

Baldock, J., Manning, N., Miller, S., Vickerstaff, S. (1999) *Social Policy*. Oxford: Oxford University Press.

Baltes, P. (1987) Theoretical propositions of life span developmental psychology: On the dynamics between growth and decline. *Developmental Psychology*, Vol. 23, No. 5, pp. 611–626.

Barn, R., Harman, V. (2006) A contested identity: An exploration of the competing social and political discourse concerning the identification and positioning of young people of inter-racial parentage. *British Journal of Social Work*, Vol. 36, No. 8, pp. 1309–1324.

Barn, R. (1999) White mothers, mixed-parentage children, and welfare. *British Journal of Social Work*, Vol. 29, No. 2, pp. 269–284.

Beattie, J. (1966) *Other Culture*. London: Routledge and Kegan Paul.

Bebbington, A., Miles, J. (1989) The background of children who enter local authority care. *British Journal of Social Work*, Vol. 19, No. 1, pp. 349–368.

Beckett, C., Maynard, A. (2005) *Values and Ethics in Social Work*. London: Sage.

Beishon, S., Modood, T., Virdee, S. (1998) *Ethnic Minority Families*. London: Policy Studies Institute.

Bennis, B. (2000) *Old Dogs, New Tricks*. London: Kogan Page.

Bernard, C., Gupta, A. (2008) Black African children and the child protection system. *British Journal of Social Work*, Vol. 38, No. 3, pp. 476–492.

Berry, J.W. (1995) Acculturative Stress, in Lonner, W.J., Malpass, R.S. (eds) *Psychology and Culture*. London: Allyn and Bacon.

Blake, R., Mouton, J. (1964) *The Managerial Grid*. Houston, TX: Gulf Publishing.

Blake, R.R., Mouton, J.S. (1981) *The Versatile Manager: A Grid Profile*. Georgetown, Ontario: Irwin-Dorsey.

Blakemore, K., Griggs, E. (2007) *Social Policy* (3rd edn). Maidenhead: McGraw Hill/Open University Press.

Borgerhoff Mulder, M., George-Cramer, M., Eshleman, J., Ortolani, A. (2001) A study of East African kinship and marriage. *American Anthropologist*, New Series, Vol. 103, No. 4, pp. 1059–1082.

Boushel, M. (2000) What kind of people are we? Race, anti-racism and social welfare research. *British Journal of Social Work*, Vol. 30, No. 1, pp. 71–89.

Brah, A. (1993) Diaspora, Border and Transnational Identities, in Lewis, R., Mills, S. (eds) *Feminist Post Colonial Theory*, Edinburgh: Edinburgh University Press.

Brechin, A., Brown, H., Eby, M.A. (2000) *Critical Practice in Health and Social Care*. London: Sage.

British Association of Social Workers (2002) Code of Ethics. Online, available at: www.basw.co.uk (accessed 17 June 2010).

Bronfenbrenner, U. (1979) *The Ecology of Human Development*. Cambridge, MA: Harvard University Press.

Brunsma, D.L. (2005) International families and the racial identification of mixed-race children: Evidence from the Early Childhood Longitudinal Study. *Social Forces*, Vol. 84, No. 2, pp. 1131–1157.

Burns, T., Stalker, G.M. (1961) *The Management of Innovation*. Oxford: Oxford University Press.

Butt, J. (2006) *Are We There Yet? Identifying the Characteristics of Social Care Organisations that Successfully Promote Diversity*. London: SCIE.

Caballero, C., Edwards, R., Puthussery, S. (2008) *Parenting Mixed Children: Negotiating Difference and Belonging in Mixed Race, Ethnicity and Faith Families*. York, UK: Joseph Rowntree Foundation.

Cameron, K. (1990) Critical questions in assessing organizational effectiveness. *Organizational Dynamics*, Autumn, pp. 66–80.

Canda, E.R. (1997) *Spirituality in Social Work: New Directions*. Binghamton, NY: Haworth Press.

Carlson, A.C. (1993) *From Cottage to Work Station: The family's Search for Social Harmony in Industrial Age*. San Francisco, CA: Ignatius Press.

Chamberlayne, P., Bornat, J., Weingref, T. (eds) (2000) *The Turn to Biographical Methods in Social Science: Comparative Issues and Example*. London: Routledge

Champayne, C., Harper Jantuah, C., Peters, J. (2007) *Different Women Different Places*. Cheam, UK: Diversity Practice Ltd.

Chand, A. (2005) Do you speak English? Language barriers in child protection social work with minority ethnic families. *British Journal of Social Work*, Vol. 35, No. 6, pp. 807–821.

Chand, A. (2008) Every child matters? A critical review of child welfare reforms in the context minority ethnic children and families. *Child Abuse Review*, Vol. 17, No. 1, pp. 6–22.

Coulshed, V., Mullender, A. (2006) Management in Social Work (3rd edn). Basingstoke, UK: Palgrave Macmillan.

Crawford, K., Walker, J. (2003) *Social Work and Human Development*. Exeter, UK: Learning Matters.

Crawford, K., Walker, J. (2007) *Social Work and Human Development* (2nd edn). Exeter, UK: Learning Matters.

Cree, V. (1995) *From Public Streets to Private Lives*. Aldershot, UK: Avebury.

Cross, W.E. (1980) Models of Psychological Nigrescence: A Literature Review, in Jones, R.L. (ed.) *Black Psychology*. New York: Harper and Row.

Cross, W.E. (1991) *Shades of Black; Diversity in African American Identity*. Philadelphia, PA: Temple University Press.

Currer, C. (2007) *Loss and Social Work*. Exeter, UK: Learning Matters.

Daley, P. (1998) Black Africans in Great Britain: Spatial concentration and segregation. *Urban Studies*, Vol. 35, No. 10, pp. 1703–1724.

Davidson, B. (1961) *Black Mother*. London: Victor Gollancz Ltd.

Davidson, B. (1984) *The Story of Africa*. London: Mitchell Beazley.

Davidson, M.J. (1997) *The Black and Ethnic Minority Woman Manager*. London: Paul Chapman.

Deacon, A. (2002) *Perspectives on Welfare*. Buckingham, UK: Open University Press.

Department of Health (2002a) *Valuing People White Paper: A strategy for Learning Disability for 21st Century*. London: Department of Health.

Department of Health (2002b) Fair Access to Care Services: Guidance on Eligibility for Adult Social Care, Local Authority Circular, LAC 13.

Department of Health (2003) *Adoption Register for England and Wales, Annual Report*. London: Adoption Register.

Diop, C.A. (1987) *Precolonial Black Africa*. Westport, CT: Lawrence Hill and Company.

Dolan, C. (2001) The 'good wife': Struggles over resources in the Kenyan horticultural sector. *Journal of Development Studies*, Vol. 37, No. 3, pp. 39–70.

Dosanjh, J.S., Ghuman, P.A.S. (1996) *Child-Rearing in Ethnic Minorities*. Clevedon: Multilingual Matters Ltd.

Drew, A. (1995) Female consciousness and feminism in Africa. *Theory and Society*, Vol. 24, No. 1, pp. 1–33.

Dubrin, A.J. (2007) *Leadership Research Findings, Practice and Skills*. Orlando, FL: Houghton Mifflin Company.

Duffy, S. (2007) Care management and self-directed support. *Journal of Integrated Care*, Vol. 15, No. 5, pp. 3–14.

Duncan, C. (2008) The dangers and limitations of equality agendas as a means for tackling old-age prejudice. *Age and Society*, Vol. 28, No. 8, pp. 1133–1158.

Dunnell, K. (2008) *Diversity and Different Experiences in the UK: National Statistician's Annual Article on Society*. London: Cabinet Office.

Eade, D. (2002) *Development and Culture*. Oxford: Oxfam.

Elam, G., Chinouya, M. (2000) *Diversity among Black African Communities*. London: National Centre for Social Research.

Ellis, J. (1978) *West African Families in Britain*. London: Routledge.

Equalities Review (2007) *Fairness and Freedom: The Final Report of the Equalities Review*. London: Cabinet Office.

Erickson, J.S. (1965) *Childhood and Society*. London: Penguin.

Evans, J.L., Myers, R.G. (1994) *Child Rearing Practices: Creating Programs Where Tradition and Modern Practices Meet*. Washington DC: Consultative Group, Notebook No. 15.

Evans, Y., Herbert, J., Datta, K. (2005) Making the city work: Low paid employment in London. Queen Mary University of London.

Fenton, S. (2003) *Ethnicity*. Cambridge, UK: Polity Press.

Ferguson, I., Lavalette, M., Mooney, G. (2002) *Rethinking Welfare: A Critical Perspective*. London: Sage.

Fernando, S. (2002) *Mental Health, Race and Culture*. Basingstoke, UK: Palgrave.

Finlay, L. (2000) The Challenge of Professionalism, in Brechin, A., Brown, H., Eby, A. (eds) *Critical Practice in Health and Social Care*. London: Sage.

Flynn, N. (1997) *Public Sector Management*. London: Harvester Press.

Frazer, L., Selwyn, J. (2005) Why are we waiting? The demography of adoption for children of black, Asian and black mixed parentage in England. *Child and Family Social Work*, Vol. 10, No. 2, pp. 135–147.

Freeman, E. (1984) *Strategic Management: A Stakeholder Approach*. London: Pitman.

Fuller, J.H.S., Toon, P.D. (1988) *Medical Practice in a Multicultural Society*. London: Heinemann.

Gabriel, Z., Bowling, A. (2004) Quality of life from the perspective of older people. *Age and Society*, Volume 24, No. 5, pp. 675–691.

Gelfand, M. (1979) *Growing Up In Shona Society*. Harare: Mambo Press.

Giddens, A. (1998) *The Third Way*. Cambridge, UK: Polity Press.

Giddens, A. (2006) *Sociology* (5th edn). Cambridge, UK: Polity Press.

Gilbert, P. (2003) *The Value of Everything*. Lyme Regis, UK: Russell House Publishing

Glasby, J. (2007) *Understanding Health and Social Care*. Bristol, UK: Social Policy Association.

Goodwin, N. (2006) *Leadership in Health Care: A European Perspective*. London: Routledge.

Gott, C., Johnston, K. (2002) The migrant population in the UK: fiscal effects. London: Home Office, RDS Occasional Paper, No. 77.

Gott, M., Seymour, J., Bellamy, G., Clark, D., Ahmedzai, S.H. (2004) Older people's views about home as a place of care at the end of life. *Palliative Medicine*, Vol. 18, No. 5, pp. 460–467.

Graham, M. (2002) *Social Work and African-Centred Worldviews*. Birmingham, UK: Venture Press.

Graham, M. (2007) Giving voice to black children: An analysis of social agency. *British Journal of Social Work*, Vol. 37, No. 8, pp. 1305–1317.

Gyimah, S.O., Tayki, B.K., Addai, I. (2006) Challenges to the reproductive-health of African women: On regional and maternal health utilization in Ghana. *Social Science and Medicine*, Vol. 62, No. 12, pp. 2930–2944.

Hall, S. (1990) Cultural Identity and Diaspora, in Rutherford, J. (ed.) *Identity Community, Culture, Difference*. London: Lawrence and Wishart.

Hall, S. (1997) *Representation: Culture Media and Identities*. London: Sage.

Handy, C. (1993) *Understanding Organizations*. London: Penguin.

Hantrais, L., Letablier, M.T. (1996) *Families and Family Policies in Europe*. London: Longman.

Harden, B. (1991) *Africa, Dispatches from a Fragile Continent*. London: Harper Collins.

Hargreaves, A., Fink, D. (2006) *Sustainable Leadership*. San Francisco, CA: Jossey-Bass.

Hatch, M.J. (1997) *Organization Theory*. Oxford: Oxford University Press.

Hatch, M.J. (2006) *Organization Theory* (2nd edn). Oxford: Oxford University Press.

Hayase, Y., Liaw, K. (1997) Factors on polygamy in Sub-Saharan Africa. *Developing Economica*, XXXV-3, pp. 293–327.

Healey, K. (2005) *Social Work Theories in Context: Creating Frameworks for Practice*. Basingstoke: Palgrave.

Henderick, H. (2003) *Child Welfare*. Bristol: Policy Press.

Holford, N.L. (1982) Religious ideation in schizophrenia. *Dissertation Abstract Journal*, Vol. 43 (6-B), 1983-B.

Holland, K., Hogg, H. (2001) *Cultural Awareness in Nursing and Health Care*. London: Arnold.

Holmes, T.H., Rahe, R.H. (1967) The social readjustment rating scale. *Journal of Psychosomatic Research*, Vol. 11, No. 2, pp. 213–318.

Horner, N. (2002) *What is Social Work: Context and Perspectives*. Exeter, UK: Learning Matters.

Huczynski, A. (2004) *Influencing Within Organizations* (2nd edn). London: Routledge.

Hugman, R. (1998) *Social Welfare and Social Value*. Basingstoke, UK: Macmillan.

Hussain, Y. Bagguley, P. (2005) Citizenship, ethnicity and identity: British Pakistanis after the 2000 'riots'. *Sociology*, Vol. 39, No. 3, pp. 407–425.

Hutson, S. (2008) Gender oppression and discrimination in South Africa. *ESSAI*, Vol. 5, Art. 26.

Ifekwunigwe, J.O. (1999) *Scattered Belongings*. London: Routledge.

IRIN (2007) International News and Analysis on Zimbabwe. Daughters fetch high price, 21 July.

Ishemo, S.L. (2002) Culture, Liberation, and Development, in Eade, D. (ed.) *Development and Culture*. Oxford: Oxfam.

Jaggar, A.M. (2005) 'Saving Amina' global justice for women and international dialogue. *Ethics and International Journal*, Vol. 19, No. 3, pp. 55–75.

James, J., Sharpley-Whiting, T.D. (2000) *The Black Feminist Reader*. Oxford: Blackwell.

Jelliffe, D.B., Bennett, F.J. (1972) Aspects of child rearing in Africa. Environmental Child Health, Monograph No. 19.

Jones, C. (2002) Social Work and Society, in Adams, R., Dominelli, L., Payne, M. (eds) *Social Work: Themes, Issues and Critical Debates*. Basingstoke, UK: Palgrave.

Kallaway, P. (2009) Education, health and social welfare in the late colonial context: The International Missionary Council and educational transition in the interwar years with specific reference to colonial Africa. *History of Education*, Vol. 38, No. 2, pp. 217–246.

Kamalu, K. (1990) *Foundations of African Thought*. London: Karnak House.

Kamara, G.M. (2000) Regaining our African aesthetics and essence through our African traditional religion. *Journal of Black Studies*, Vol. 30, No. 4, pp. 502–514.

Karenga, M. (1993) *Introduction to Black Studies* (2nd edn). Los Angeles, CA: University of Sankore Press.

Kaseke, E. (1999) Social Security and the Elderly, *Courier* No. 76, pp. 50–52.

Kemshall, H. (2002) *Risk, Social Policy and Welfare*. Buckingham, UK: Open University Press.

Kevane, M. (2004) *Women and Development in Africa*. London: Lynne Rienner.

Killingray, D. (1994) *Africans in Britain*. London: Cass and Co.

Kim, C.H., Draper, J. (2008) *Liberating Texts?* London: SPCK.

Koenig, M.A., Tulalo, T., Zhao, F., Nalugoda, F. (2003) Domestic violence in rural Uganda: Evidence from a community based study. *Bulletin of the World Health Organization*, Vol. 81, No. 1, pp. 53–60.

Kohli, R.K.S. (2006) The comfort of strangers: Social work practice with unaccompanied asylum-seeking children and young people in the UK. *Child and Family Social Work*, Vol. 11, No. 1, pp. 1–10.

Kyambi, S. (2005) *Beyond Black and White: Mapping New Immigrant Communities*. London: IPPR.

Laming, H. (2003) *Enquiry Report into the Death of Victoria Climbie*. London: The Stationery Office.

Laming, H. (2009) *The Protection of Children in England: A Progress Report*. London: The Stationery Office.

Lawler, J., Bilson, A. (2010) *Social Work Management and Leadership*. Oxford, UK: Routledge.

Lawrence, P.R., Lorsch, J.W. (1967) *Organization and Environment*. Cambridge, MA: Harvard University Press.

Leslie, G.R. (1982) *The Family in Social Context* (5th edn). Oxford: Oxford University Press.

Lester, N.A. (2000) Nappy edges and goldy locks: African American daughters and the politics of hair. *Lion and the Unicorn*, Vol. 24, No. 2, pp. 201–224.

Lewin, K. (1947) Frontiers in group dynamics: Concept, method and reality in social science; social equilibria and social change. *Human Relations*, Vol. 1, No. 1, pp. 5–41.

Lewis, G., Gewitz, S., Clarke, J. (2000) *Rethinking Social Policy*. London: Sage.

Llewellyn, A., Agu, L., Mercer, D. (2008) *Sociology for Social Workers*. Cambridge, UK: Polity Press.

Loewenthal, K.M., Cinnrelli, M. (2003) Religious Issues in Ethnic Minority Mental Health, in Ndegwa, D., Olajide, D. (eds) *Main Issues in Mental Health and Race*. Aldershot, UK: Ashgate.

Logan, S.L. (1996) *The Black Family: Strengths Self-help and Positive Change*. Oxford, UK: Westview Press.

Louw, B., Avenant, C. (2002) Culture as context for intervention: Developing a culturally congruent early intervention program. *International Pediatrics*, Vol. 17, No. 3, pp. 145–150.

Lymberry, M., Postle, K. (2007) *Social Work: A Companion to Learning*. London: Sage.

Lyons, K., Manion, K., Carlsen, M. (2006) *International Perspective on Social Work*. Basingstoke, UK: Palgrave Macmillan.

McAdoo, H.P. (1988) *Black Families* (2nd edn). London: Sage.

Mckimm, J., Phillips, K. (2009) *Leadership and Management in Integrated Services*. Exeter, UK: Learning Matters.

Mann, K. (1984) The dangers of dependence: Christian marriage among elite women in Lagos. *Journal of African History*, Vol. 24, No. 1, pp. 37–57.

Manor, O. (2000) *Choosing a Groupwork Approach: An Inclusive Stance*. London: Jessica Kingsley.

Maringe, F., Lumby, J., Morrison, M., Bhopal, K., Dyke, M. (2007) *Leadership, Diversity and Decision Making*. Lancaster, UK: Centre for Excellence in Leadership.

Marshall, T.H. (1950) *Citizenship and Social Class*. London: Heinemann.

Mathabane, M. (1994) *African Women, Three Generations*. London: Hamish Hamilton.

Martin, V., Henderson, E. (2001) *Managing in Health and Social Care*. London: Routledge.

Maxime, J.E. (1993) Some Psychological Models of Black Self-concept, in Ahmed, S., Cheetham, J., Small, J. (eds) *Social Work with Black Children and their Families*. London: Batsford.

Mbiti, J. (1970) *Africans Religions and Philosophy*. Garden City, NY: Anchor Books.

Meekers, D. (1992) The process of marriage in African societies. *Population and Development Review*, Vol. 18, No. 1, pp. 61–78.

Miller, S. (2006) *Counselling Skills for Social Work*. London: Sage.

Mintzberg, H. (1973) *The Nature of Managerial Work*. New York: Harper and Row.

Moghaddam, F.M. (1998) *Social Psychology: Exploring Universals Across Cultures*. New York: Freeman and Company.

Moller Okin, S. (1994) Gender inequality and cultural differences. *Political Theory*, Vol. 22, No. 1, pp. 5–24.

Moriarty, J., Butt, J. (2004) Inequalities in quality of life among people from different ethnic groups. *Age and Society*, Vol. 24, No. 5, pp. 729–753.

Moyo, D. (2010) *Dead Aid*. London: Penguin.

Mvududu, S., McFadden, P. (2001) *Reconceptualizing the Family in a Changing Southern African Environment*. Harare: WLSA.

Nangoli, M. (1986) *No More Lies About Africa*. New Jersey: African Heritage Publishers.

Newman, J. (2000) Beyond the New Public Management? Modernizing Public Services, in Clarke, J., Gewirtz, S., McLaughlin, E. (eds) *New Managerialism New Welfare*. London: Sage.

Nkomo, S., Cox, T. (1996) Diverse Identities in Organizations, in Clegg, S., Hardy, C., Nord, W. (eds) *Managing Organizations: Current Issues*. London: Sage.

Nzira, V. Williams, P. (2009) *Anti-Oppressive Practice in Health and Social Care*. London: Sage.

O'Brien, M., Penna, S. (1998) *Theorising Welfare: Enlightenment and Modern Society*. London: Sage.

Oakley, A. (2000) *Experiments in Knowing*. Cambridge, UK: Polity Press.

Obbo, C. (1980) *African Women: Their Struggle for Economic Independence*. London: Zed Press.

Obomanu, W. (2003) Black Families, in Ndegwa, D., Olajide, D. (eds) *Main Issues in Mental Health and Race*. Aldershot: Ashgate.

Oguibe, O. (1994) *Sojourners: New Writings by Africans in Britain*. London: Refugee Publishing Collective.

Okitikpi, T., Aymer, C. (2003) Social care with African families and their children. *Child and Family Social Work*, Vol. 8, No. 3, pp. 213–222.

Oko, J. (2008) *Understanding and Using Theory in Social Work*. Exeter, UK: Learning Matters.

Olumide, G. (2005) Mixed Race Children: Policy and Practice Consideration, in Okitikpi, T. (ed.) *Working with Children of Mixed Parentage*. Lyme Regis, UK: Russell House Publishing.

Olusanya, B., Hodes, D. (2000) West African children in private foster care. *Child Care Health and Development*, Vol. 26, No. 4, pp. 337–342.

Owen, M. (1996) *A World Of Widows*. London: Zed Books.

Paludi, M.A. (2002) *Human Development in Multi-Cultural Context: A Book of Readings*. Upper Saddle River, NJ: Prentice Hall.

Parker, P.S. (2005) *Race, Gender, and Leadership*. London: Lawrence Erlbaum.

Parks, S. (2001) In My Mother's House: Black Feminist Aesthetics, Television and A Raisin in the Sun, in Bobo, J. (ed.) *Black Feminist Cultural Criticism*. Oxford: Blackwell.

Patel, V., Mutambirwa, J., Nhiwatiwa, S. (2002) Stressed, Depressed, or Bewitched? A Perspective on Mental Health, Culture and Religion, in Eade, D. (ed.) *Development and Culture*. Oxford: Oxfam.

Pettinger, R. (2000) *Mastering Organisational Behaviour*. Basingstoke, UK: Palgrave.

Pierce, L., Bozalek, V. (2004) Child abuse in South Africa: An examination of how child abuse and neglect are defined. *Child Abuse and Neglect*, Vol. 28, No. 8, pp. 817–832.

Population Reference Bureau and African Population Research Centre (2008) African Population Data Sheet (2), Washington and Nairobi PRB and APHRC.

Powell, M. (2000) New Labour and the third way in the British welfare state: A new and distinctive approach? *Critical Social Policy*, Vol. 20, No. 1, pp. 39–60.

Powell, M., Hewitt, M. (2002) *Welfare State and Welfare Change*. Buckingham, UK: Open University Press.

Pugh, D.S., Hickson, D.J. (1996) *Writer On Organizations* (5th edn). London: Penguin.

Rahim, M.A. (2002) Towards a theory of managing conflict. *International Journal of Conflict Management*, Vol. 13, No. 3, pp. 206–235.

Ranger, T. (1986) Religious movements and politics in Sub-Saharan Africa. *African Studies Review*, Vol. 29, No. 2, pp. 2–69.

Ranger, T. (1995) *Are We Not Also Men?* London: James Currey.

Rapoport, R., Rapoport, R.N. (1975) *Leisure and the family cycle*. London: Routledge.

Ridge, D., Williams, I., Anderson, J., Elford, J. (2008) Like a prayer: The role of spirituality and religion for people living with HIV in the UK. *Sociology of Health and Illness*, Vol. 30, No. 3, pp. 413–428.

Roakeach, M. (1973) *The Nature of Human Values*. New York: Free Press.

Robinson, L. (2000) Racial identity attitudes and self-esteem of black adolescents in residential care: An exploratory study. *British Journal of Social Work*, Vol. 30, No. 1, pp. 3–24.

Rowntree, B.S. (1901) A Study of Town Life. London: Macmillan.

Ruth, S. (2006) Leadership and Liberation. London: Routledge.

Saleebey, D. (2002) *The Strength Perspective in Social Work Practice* (3rd edn). London: Allyn and Bacon.

SARDC-WIDSAA (2000) *Beyond Inequalities: Women in Southern Africa*. Harare: SARDC.

Schein, E.H. (2004) *Organizational Culture and Leadership* (3rd edn). San Francisco, CA: Jossey-Bass.

Schroder-Butterfill, E., Marianti, R. (2006) A framework for understanding old-age vulnerabilities. *Age and Society*, Vol. 26, No. 1, pp. 9–35.

Schwarz-Bart, S. (2003) *In Praise of Black Women*. Madison, WI: University of Wisconsin Press.

SCIE (2004) Position Paper No. 3: Has service user participation made a difference to social care services? London: SCIE. Online, available at: http://www.scie.org.uk (accessed 17 June 2010).

SCIE (2008) *Has Service User Participation Made a Difference to Social Care Services?* London: SCIE.

Scott, W.R. (2001) *Institutions and Organizations* (2nd edn). London: Sage.

Scottish Leadership Foundation (2005) *21st Century Social Work*. Edinburgh: Scottish Executive.

Seden, J., Ross, T. (2007) Active Service User Involvement in Human Services: Lessons From Practice, in Aldgate, J., Healy, L., Malcolm, B., Pine, B. (eds) *Enhancing Social Work Management*. London: Jessica Kingsley.

Sentamu, J. (2008) Uncovering the Purposes of God, in Kim, S.C.H., Draper, J. (eds) *Liberating Texts? Sacred Scriptures in Public Life*. London: SPCK.

Sharkey, P. (2007) *The Essentials of Community Care*. Basingstoke, UK: Palgrave Macmillan.

Sheldon, B., Macdonald, G. (2009) *A Textbook of Social Work*. London: Routledge.

Siddiqui, A. (2008) Text and Context: Making Sense of Islam in the Modern World, in Kim, S.C.H., Draper, J. (eds) *Liberating Texts? Sacred Scriptures in Public Life*. London: SPCK.

Small, J. (1993) Transracial Placements: Conflict and Contradictions, in Ahmed, S., Cheetham, J., Small, J. (eds) *Social Work with Black Children and Their Families*. London: Batsford.

Snyder, M. (2000) *Women in African Economics*. Kampala: Fountain Publishers.

Social Services Inspectorate (2002) *A Joint Chief Inspectors Report on Safeguarding Children*. London: SSI.

Social Work Task Force (2009) *Final Report: Building a Safe and Confident Future*. London: Cabinet Office. Online, available at: http:publications.dcsf.gov.uk (accessed 17 June 2010).

Stacey, J., Meadow, T. (2009) New slants on the slippery slope: The politics of polygamy and gay family rights in South Africa and the United States. *Politics and Society*, Vol. 37, No. 2, pp. 167–202.

Stuart, S. (1996) Female-headed families: A comparative perspective of the Caribbean and the developed world. *Gender and Development*, Vol. 4, No. 2, pp. 28–34.

Sue, D.W., Carter, R.T., Orredondo, J.R. (1998) *Multicultural Counselling Competences*. London: Sage.

Takyi, B.K. (2003) Religion and women's health in Ghana: Insights into HIV/AIDs preventive and protective behaviour. *Social Science and Medicine*, Vol. 56, No. 6, pp. 1221–1234.

Taylor, A.M. (2003) *Responding to Adolescents*. Lyme Regis, UK: RHP.

Thiam, A. (1986) *Black Sisters Speak Out*. London: Pluto Press.

Thoburn, J., Chand, A., Procter, J. (2005) *Child Welfare Services for Minority Ethnic Families*. London: Jessica Kingsley.

Tizard, B., Phoenix, A. (1993) *Black, White or Mixed Race*. London: Routledge.

United Nations (2005) *The Millennium Development Goals: Progress Report*. New York: United Nations.

Ver Beek, K.L. (2002) Spirituality: A Development Taboo, in Eade, D. (ed.) *Development and Culture*, Oxford: Oxfam.

Ward, D. (2002) Groupwork, in Adam, R., Dominelli, L., Payne, M. (eds) *Social Work Themes, Issues and Critical Debates*. Basingstoke, UK: Palgrave.

Warren, K. (2003) *Exploring the Concept of Recovery from the Perspective of People with Mental Health Problems*. Norwich, UK: Social Work Monographs.

Weber, M. (1947) *The Theory of Social and Economic Organization*. New York: Free Press.

Williams, F. (1995) Race/ethnicity, gender, and class in welfare states: A framework for comparative analysis. *Social Politics*, Vol. 2, No. 2, pp. 127–159.

Williams, F. (2001) In and beyond New Labour: towards a political ethics of care. *Critical Social Policy*, Vol. 21, No. 4, pp. 467–493.

Williams, F. (2002) The presence of feminism in the future of welfare. *Economy and Society*, Vol. 31, No, 4, pp. 503–518.

WLSA (2000) *In The Shadow of the Law*. Harare: WLSA.

Index

UNIVERSITY OF WINCHESTER
LIBRARY